Universal Health Coverage

Edited by Aida Isabel Tavares

Published in London, United Kingdom

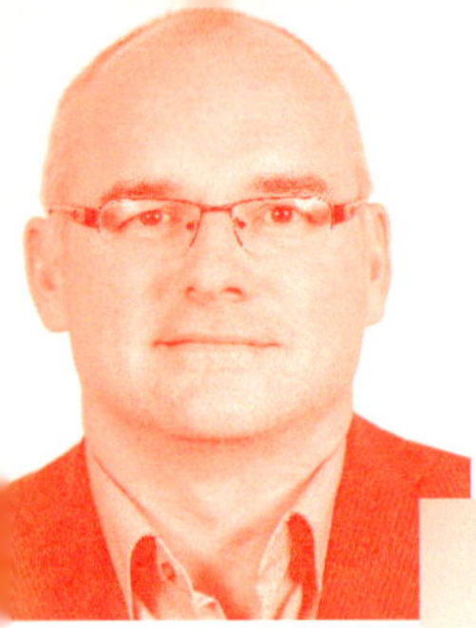
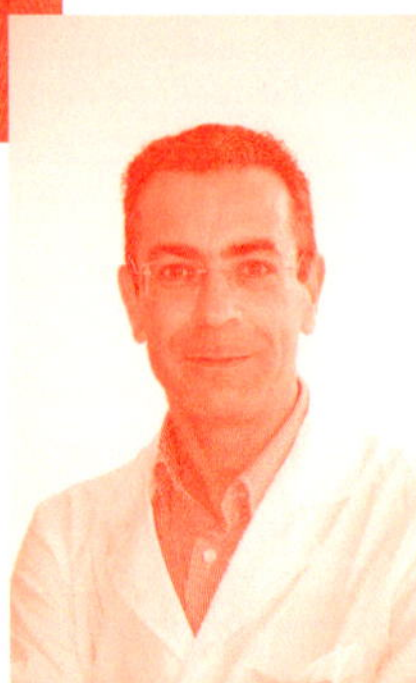
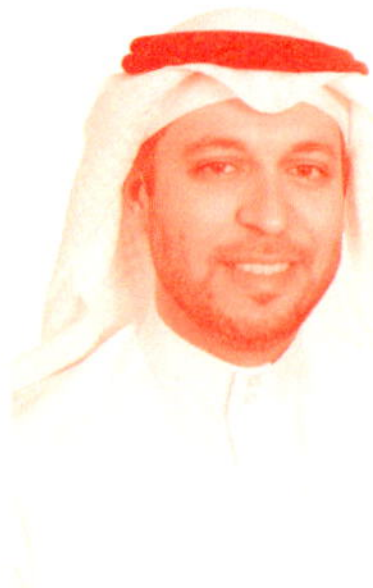
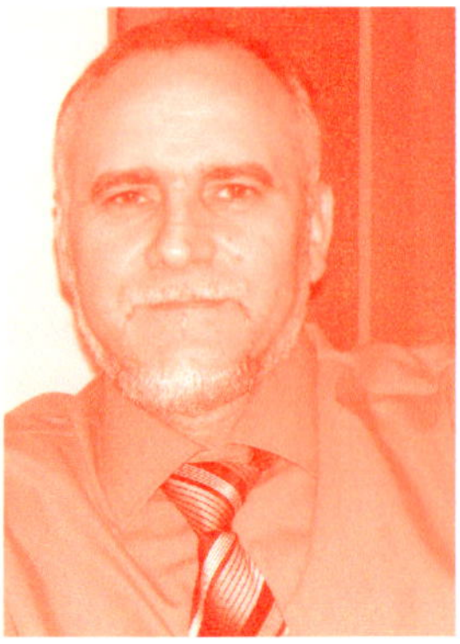
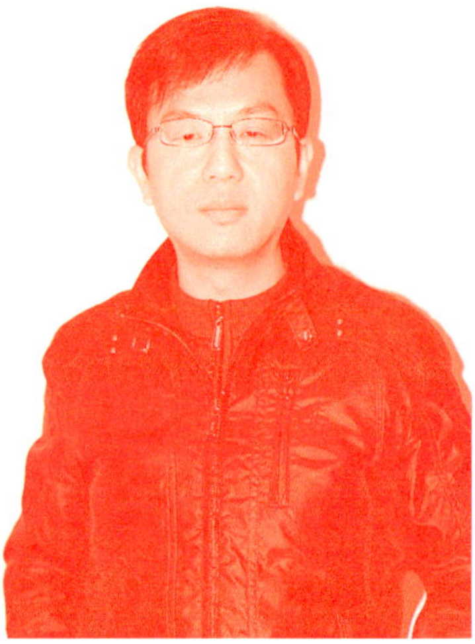
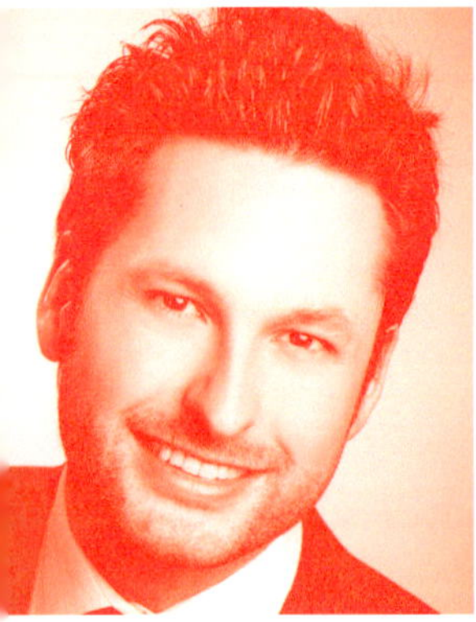
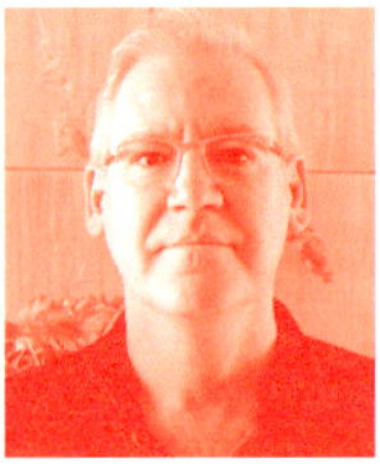

IntechOpen

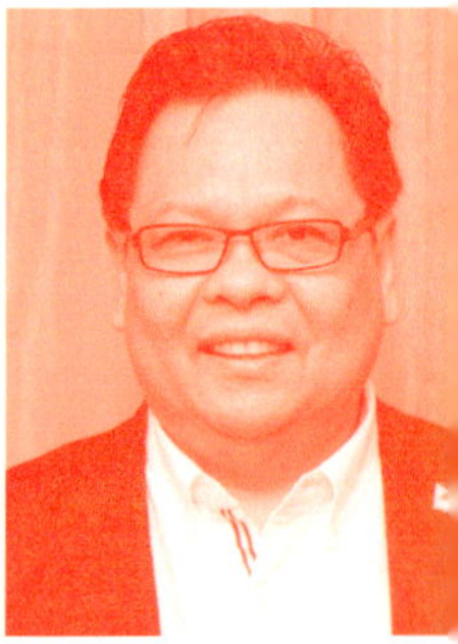
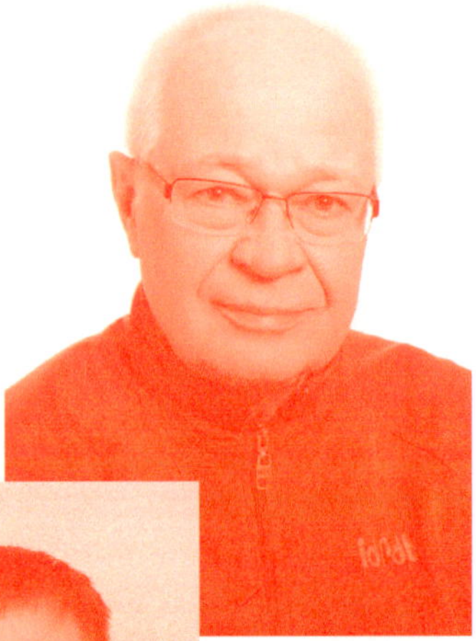
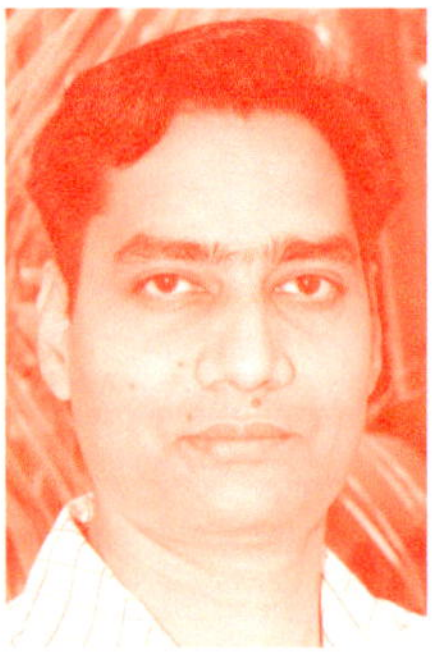
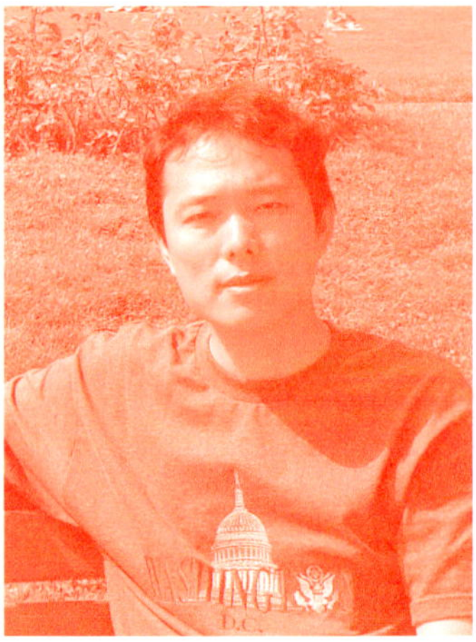
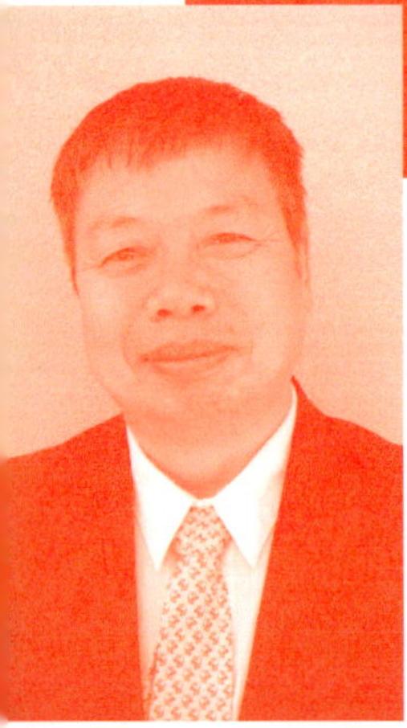
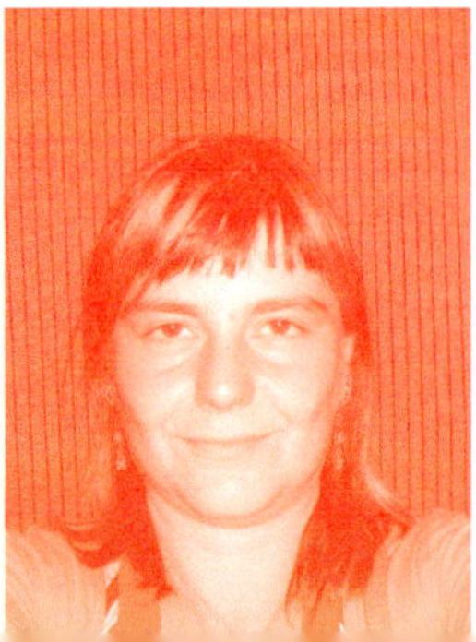

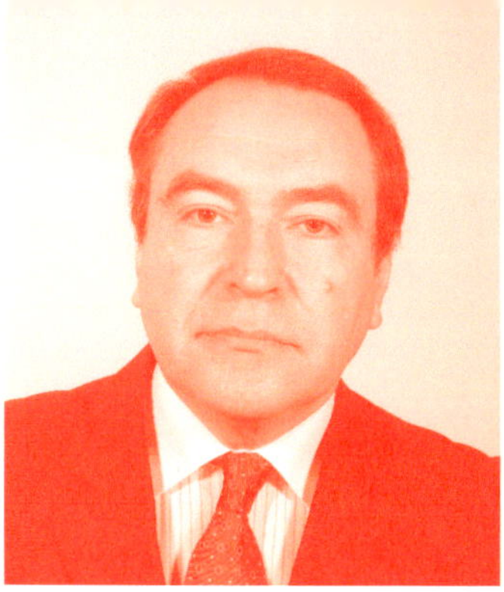

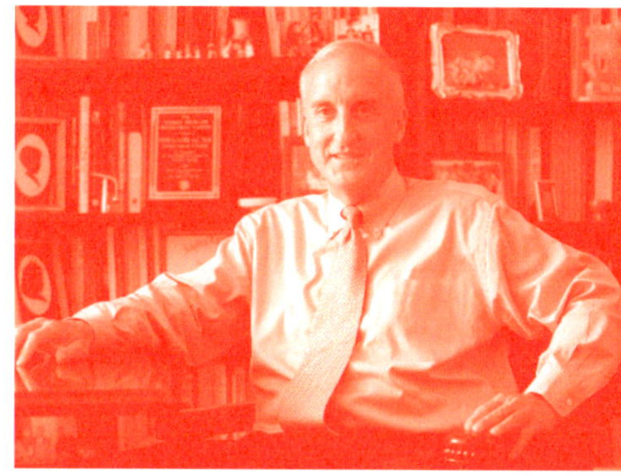

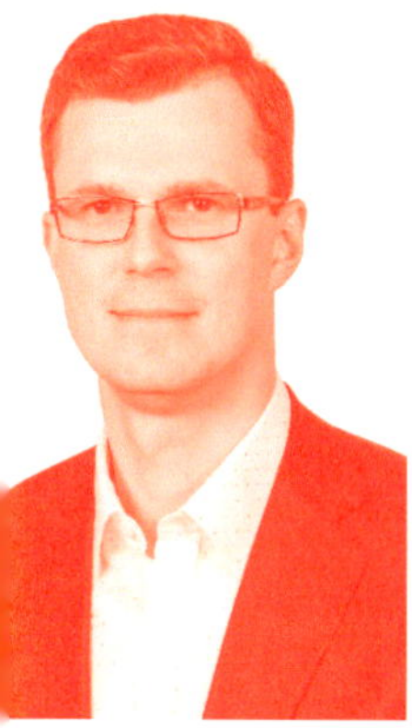

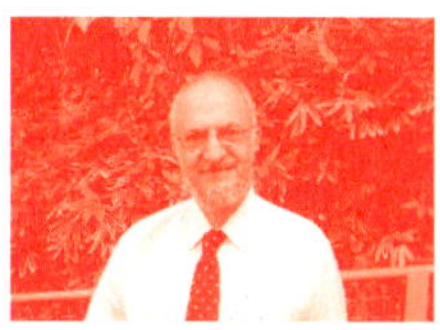

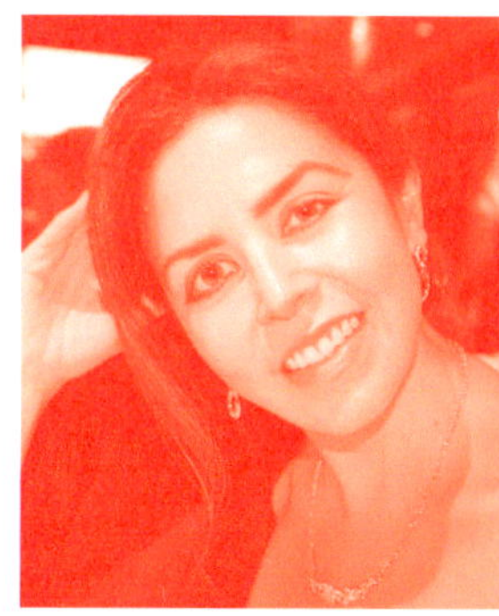

Supporting open minds since 2005

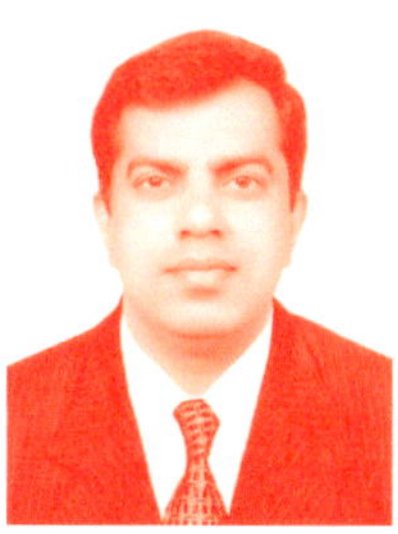

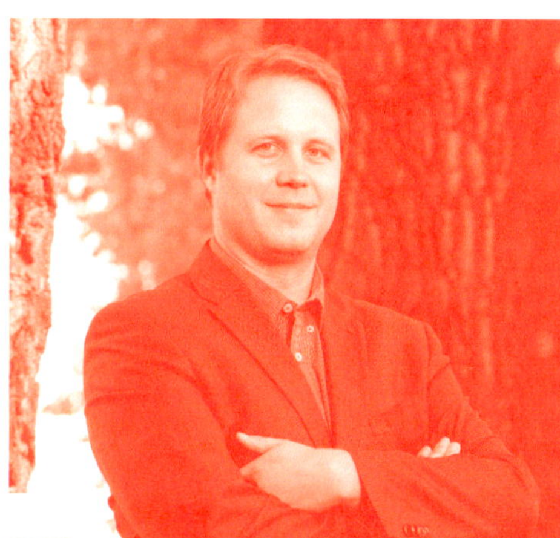

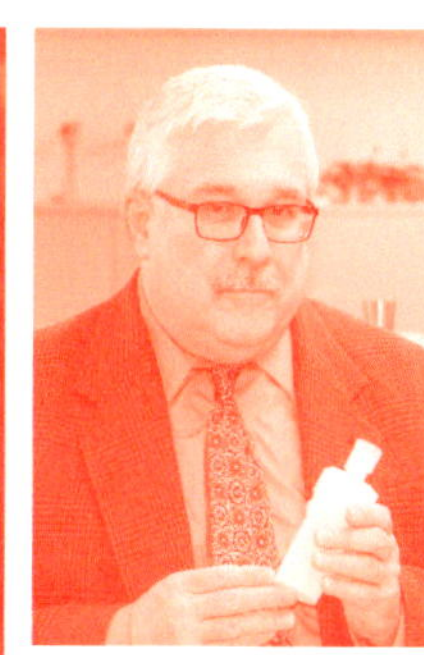

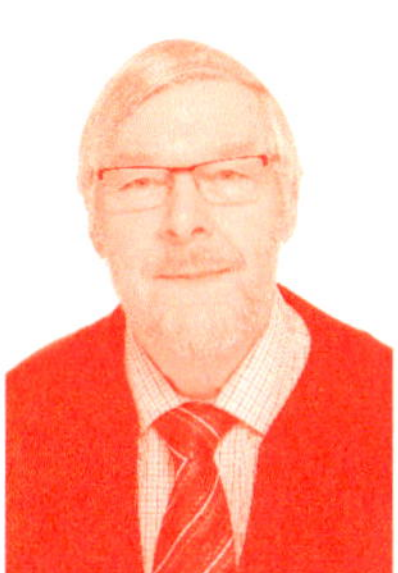

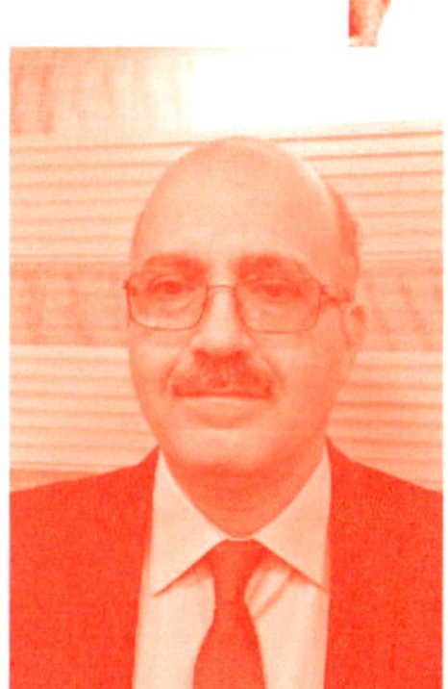

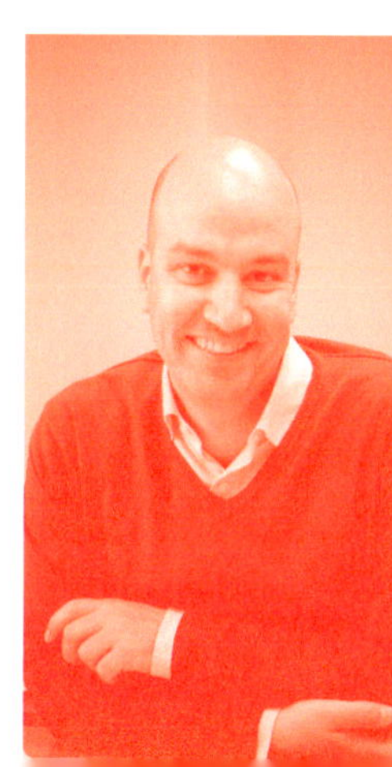

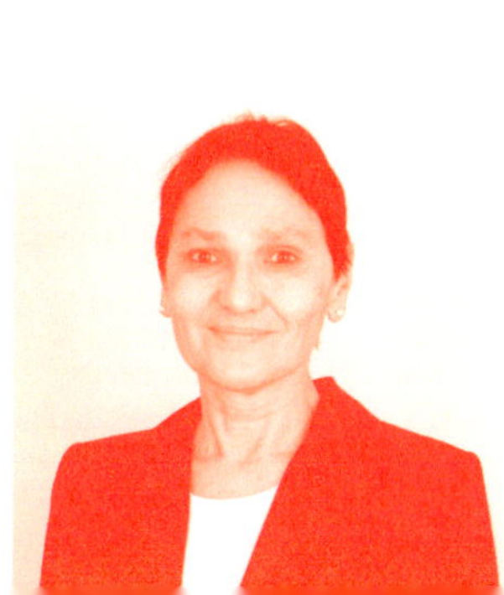

Universal Health Coverage
http://dx.doi.org/10.5772/intechopen.77664
Edited by Aida Isabel Tavares

Contributors
Lorena Saletti-Cuesta, Lila Aizenberg, Alex Asakitikpi, Sandra Pennbrant, Margareta Karlsson, Abualbishr Alshreef, Stefano Neri, Telma Maria Menicucci, Aida Isabel Tavares

First published in London, United Kingdom, 2019 by IntechOpen
IntechOpen is the global imprint of INTECHOPEN LIMITED, registered in England and Wales, registration number: 11086078, 7th floor, 10 Lower Thames Street, London, EC3R 6AF, United Kingdom
Printed in Croatia

British Library Cataloguing-in-Publication Data
A catalogue record for this book is available from the British Library

Additional hard and PDF copies can be obtained from orders@intechopen.com

Universal Health Coverage
Edited by Aida Isabel Tavares
p. cm.
Print ISBN 978-1-78984-974-5
Online ISBN 978-1-78984-975-2
eBook (PDF) ISBN 978-1-78984-646-1

For EU product safety concerns:
IN TECH d.o.o., Prolaz Marije Krucifikse Kozulić 3, 51000 Rijeka, Croatia, info@intechopen.com or visit our website at intechopen.com.

Meet the editor

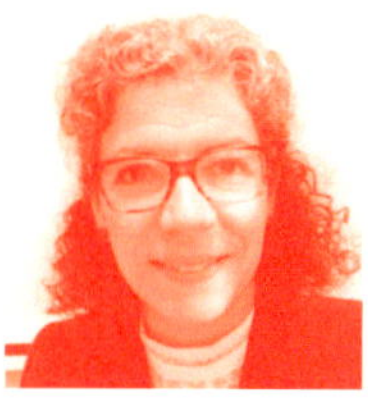

Aida Isabel Tavares holds a PhD in Economic Analysis awarded by the Autónoma University of Barcelona in 2008. Her research focus has been on health economics, policy and management and she has published several articles in international peer-reviewed journals. She has also published a book on public economics. Prof. Tavares has been teaching several courses, at different universities, including microeconomics, health economics and public economics. Currently she collaborates with the Centre of Studies and Research in Health at the University of Coimbra and she is an Assistant Professor in the Lisbon School of Economics and Management, University of Lisbon.

Contents

Preface

Universal health coverage (UHC) is a major ambition of every health system in the world. It advocates that quality health services are to be accessed by all people, when needed, without being too expensive. This ambition has been clearly stated as a target for the Sustainable Development Goal defined by the United Nations in the UN Millennium Summit of 2000. The World Health Organization in 2013 published the 'World Health Report: Research for universal health coverage', which presented the importance of researching and discussing how to achieve universal health coverage. The main purpose of this book is contributing to the ongoing discussion on this topic.

This book starts with the chapter "Funding Universal Healthcare and Long-Term Care in an Aging Era" by Aida Isabel Tavares and Pedro Lopes Ferreira, where the concept of UHC is described as well as the funding of UHC and long-term care in the demographic scenario of aging. This chapter details several introductory concepts on UHC and relates them with LTC in aging societies.

Under the topic of funding, Abualbishr Alshreef wrote the next chapter "Provider Payment Mechanisms: Effective Policy Tools for Achieving Universal and Sustainable Healthcare Coverage". One role of funding UHC is paying providers for the healthcare services supplied to people. The payment mechanism needs to be strategic in order to promote cost containment. This chapter reviews the problem of increasing cost in health services in low- and middle-income countries and explores the alternative payment mechanisms which may contain the rising costs and which may contribute to the implementation of UHC.

Funding is fundamental to ensure that UHC may be achieved and this includes the prevention of catastrophic health expenditures or financial hardship. The next chapter "Healthcare Coverage and Affordability in Nigeria: An Alternative Model to Equitable Healthcare Delivery" by Alex Asakitikpi addressed this topic. In Nigeria there have been several efforts to promote health equity and guarantee of access to all citizens; however, the results are worse than expected. The authors propose measures related to provider's payments that are all-embracing towards the provision of healthcare services to Nigerians and other low- and medium-income countries.

UHC foresees access to quality healthcare services. Sandra Pennbrant in the next chapter "Caring for Older Persons - Improving Healthcare Quality to Ensure Well-being and Dignity" discusses the importance of treating the elderly with dignity and a caring attitude and how this can be done. This is particularly important in a world where the aging phenomenon is changing the demographic structure.

The concern for quality continues in the next chapter entitled "An Intersectional Innovative Analysis of How Providers' Discourses Interacts with Universal Healthcare Access" by Lorena Saletti-Cuesta. Focusing on Argentina, the author explores how the intersectionality may help to understand the multiple axes of inequalities that cross healthcare providers' discourses on violence against women and health problems of migrant women.

The two last chapters of this book present the evolution of UHC in two very different countries: Brazil, a medium income country, and Italy, a European developed country.

The Brazilian case is presented by Telma Maria Menicucci and it focuses on the implementation of a universal health system. The chapter describes the last 30 years of history, the successes and the difficulties of implementing such health system in a large developing country. At the end of this chapter, the author highlights the challenges that are emerging in the Brazilian health system.

The Italian case is portrayed by Stefano Neri. This country has faced an economic crisis for the last 10 years and the negative impacts on the National Health System are now observable. Quality has suffered as well as access to healthcare services. The emerging social and territorial inequalities weaken the universalistic nature of the Italian Health System.

Aida Isabel Tavares
Lisbon School of Economics and Management,
University of Lisbon,
Lisbon, Portugal

Centre of Studies and Research in Health,
University of Coimbra,
Coimbra, Portugal

Section 1

Introduction

Chapter 1

Introductory Chapter: Universal Health Coverage

Aida Isabel Tavares

1. Introduction

Universal health coverage (UHC) is a major ambition of every health system around the world. It stands for the aspiration that health services are to be accessed by all people, when needed with quality, without falling in financial debt or bankruptcy. This ambition has been clearly stated as a target for the Sustainable Development Goal defined by the United Nations in the UN Millennium Summit of 2000. The World Health Organisation (WHO), in 2013, published the 'World health report: research for universal health coverage' [1] where it becomes evident the importance of researching and discussing how to advance towards universal health coverage. The main purpose of this book is contributing to the ongoing discussion on this topic.

2. Universal health coverage

Universal health coverage conveys an ambitious idea of ensuring health care services of quality to all people who are in need, without suffering financial hardship. According to the latest UHC monitoring by WHO, in 2017 [2], this goal is still a bit far away from what was defined initially. About 100 million of people in the world fall into extreme poverty because of out-of-pocket expenditures. Almost 180 million of people spend 25% or more of the household budget on health expenditures, and this figure has been rising for about 5% each year globally.

These astonishing numbers slowdown the movement towards the Sustainable Development Goals (SDG) [3], both the SDG1—ending poverty and the SDG3—ensuring healthy lives and promoting well-being. This later SDG includes Target 3.8 which is concerned precisely with the achievement of UHC. The importance of UHC has been recognised by governments, who have in several occasions committed moving towards UHC. Regardless numbers, there are good news. The latest report on monitoring UHC worldwide concluded that there has been some progress towards UHC despite the unequal and slow speed of improvement.

The measurement of the movement towards UHC is based on three dimensions [1]: (i) who is covered, (ii) which services are covered and (iii) how much cost is covered. The first dimension measures the proportion of people who is covered and the aim is 100%. The second dimension measures the number and type of services to be supplied to people. The third dimension measures the cost-sharing of accessing to health services between people and the health system. The role of governments is then (i) to decide which are the health services to be included in the package of services and the quality of the services, and (ii) to ensure that people have access to these services in affordable way. This decision is different across countries and across time. It depends on several variables such as economic development, available technology, climate and epidemiology features.

3. Investing in universal health coverage

Investing in UHC is to have a stake in each country health system. The meaning of investing is wide and the impacts can also be wide, either immediate or medium and long-run impacts on the health system and population health.

The inputs of UHC where governments may invest include financing, producing health workforce, investing in medicines and infrastructures, as well as in information, and also creating a well-adjusted governance structure.

The immediate impact of these inputs is felt on the provision of services. Health services are expected to account for access, readiness, quality and safety. Inputs also allow for creating a financial pool needed to support UHC. The non-immediate impacts of investing in UHC happen on the desired outcomes. These are, in fact, the three dimensions used to measure the progress of UHC meaning coverage, financial risk protection and risk dispersion. The final and long-lasting impact is felt by the population: the improved health status and financial well-being, and by the health system itself: the increased responsiveness and health security.

Along the different stages of this chain of inputs and impacts, the social determinants are a permanent influence to be considered to ensure equity of coverage. At the end, from an overall view, investing and providing UHC implies producing health services in quantity and quality and in equitable base.

With this framework in mind, one realises that the research and analysis on the improvement of UHC is diversified and addresses several topics and issues, from the inputs, to the outputs and outcomes, ending at the population health, and going through social determinants, quality and equity. The ground for studying UHC is vast.

This book contributes to the discussion on the universal health coverage and no single topic is privileged. The main aim here is to joint different perspectives and contributions on how to improve UHC. The variety of topics presented and discussed along the book confirms the importance that UHC has for academics and health professionals. But it also remarks the controversies and challenges of its implementation and improvement.

4. Invitation

The reader is invited to read about a variety of topics emerging in the context of universal health coverage around the world and be involved in some of the current discussions.

Author details

Aida Isabel Tavares[1,2]

1 Lisbon School of Economics and Management, University of Lisbon, Lisbon, Portugal

2 Centre of Studies and Research in Health, University of Coimbra, Coimbra, Portugal

*Address all correspondence to: aitavar@gmail.com

References

[1] WHO. The World Health Report 2013: Research for Universal Coverage. Geneva: WHO; 2013

[2] WHO. Tacking Universal Health Coverage: 2017 Global Monitoring Report. World Health Organization and the International Bank for Reconstruction and Development / The World Bank; 2017

[3] UN. Sustainable Development Goals. 2019. Available at https://sustainabledevelopment.un.org/topics/sustainabledevelopmentgoals

Section 2

Funding

Chapter 2

Provider Payment Mechanisms: Effective Policy Tools for Achieving Universal and Sustainable Healthcare Coverage

Abualbishr Alshreef

Abstract

Globally, governments are seeking to develop equitable and sustainable healthcare systems for delivering universal healthcare coverage under budget constraints. This chapter provides an analysis of fee-for-service, a commonly used payment mechanism for reimbursement of healthcare providers, and proposes appropriate reform in order to promote cost containment in the context of low- and middle-income countries (LMICs). The analysis used secondary data derived from the literature. The analysis revealed that capitation, case-based, and global budget provider payment mechanisms have the potential to control healthcare costs by creating incentives for providers to reduce the volume of services. Capitation payment has the potential to promote provider efficiency, while global budget may reward inefficient hospitals if risk adjustors (such as gender and age) are not considered in the resource allocation formula. Both capitation payment and global budget have lower administrative costs compared to fee-for-service. Development of supporting measures is crucial including legal, financial, referral, quality assurance, and management information systems.

Keywords: health reforms, funding, health insurance, provider payment, expenditure and costs, cost containment, LMICs

1. Introduction

Healthcare provider payment mechanisms can be used as powerful tools for promoting the development of health systems towards the achievement of health policy objectives by encouraging the effective and efficient use of scarce resources [1]. This chapter provides an in-depth review addressing the problem of the escalating costs of health services for low- and middle-income countries (LMIC) and explores alternative provider payment mechanisms for promoting cost containment and contributes to universal and sustainable healthcare coverage. This introduction section provides background information with more focus on the widely used fee-for-service (FFS) provider payment mechanism and its impact on healthcare costs.

During the past four decades, the escalation of healthcare costs for LMICs has been an issue of concern at both operational and policy levels. Many policy tools

IntechOpen

have been implemented to control the escalation in cost and/or to absorb its negative effect in many countries. This included revenue generation through the expansion of health insurance population coverage, strengthening contracting capacity, and reimbursement of pharmaceuticals based on essential medicines lists (EMLs). However, the cost of health services has remained a big challenge for healthcare systems in many LMICs.

As an alternative strategic approach, provider payment mechanisms can create incentives for wise and efficient use of resources and create a behavioural environment for healthcare providers to supply cost-effective health services [1–3]. By exploring alternative provider payment mechanisms and assessing their effect in controlling healthcare costs, potentially feasible measures based on good quality evidence may be proposed. Providing evidence for provider payment reform is strategically important to contribute to the decision-making process to tackle the increasing costs of health services for LMICs. This will contribute to the ongoing reforms towards universal healthcare coverage in many countries.

This chapter analyses the existing provider payment mechanism (widely used in LMIC context) and proposes payment system reform in order to promote cost containment. A conceptual framework was used to analyse the existing provider payment mechanism, explore alternative mechanisms and assess their potential in promoting cost containment in LMICs. The chapter identifies lessons learned from international experiences on cost containment for health insurance schemes (and similar funding structures) and assesses the most appropriate options. The feasibility of implementing the proposed cost containment measures in the context of LMICs is discussed.

This chapter is structured into five sections starting with this introductory section. Then, Section 2 describes the methodology and conceptual framework used for the analysis. Section 3 analyses the problem of the escalating costs of health services in LMIC context and uses the conceptual framework for the analysis of the existing FFS payment. Section 4 then analyses the alternative provider payment mechanisms for controlling healthcare cost using the same conceptual framework. Finally, Section 5 is a concluding section, summarises the key messages, suggests potential measures emerged from the analysis and assesses the feasibility of implementing the proposed reform in LMICs.

This chapter of the book is primarily intended for use by policymakers to contribute as evidence in the decision-making process for strategic purchasing of health services in LMIC context. The evidence provided would also be useful for researchers interested in healthcare financing and for other health insurance organisations in LMICs. Furthermore, international development partners interested in health insurance in LMICs may also be interested in this review, including World Bank (WB), International Labour Organisation (ILO) and World Health Organisation (WHO).

2. Conceptual framework, data and limitations of the review

Having addressed the background information and the aim of the review in the previous section, this section describes the conceptual framework used for the analysis, sources of data and the limitations of the review. This chapter of the book provides an in-depth review exploring alternative healthcare provider-payment mechanisms particularly capitation, case-based and global budget as potential policy tools for use in the LMICs. The review is based on secondary data from the literature combined with the author's 8 years of experience in LMIC context.

2.1 The conceptual framework

The conceptual framework used was adapted from the literature, bearing in mind a basic question: *"how provider payment mechanisms work to control healthcare costs?"*. The framework is schematically represented in **Figure 1**. It was developed to articulate the analysis of provider payment mechanisms presented in this chapter.

2.1.1 Description of the conceptual framework

The conceptual framework illustrated in **Figure 1** is composed of three columns, which are clearly distinguished by different colours and these columns are interlinked by arrows to demonstrate conceptual relationships. The yellow column on the left side represents four provider payment mechanisms: the FFS currently used in many LMICs and the three alternative payment mechanisms explored in this review (capitation, case-based and global budget). The yellow arrows are pointing to the key output aspects outlined in the middle purple column.

The middle purple column illustrates the processes that affect each payment mechanism and, therefore, impact on the cost of health services [4]. Provider payment mechanisms work by creating incentives that affect the volume of supplied services, use of input resources, pharmaceuticals, admission rate, average length of stay and prevention of diseases [1, 4]. Administrative cost varies between the different payment mechanisms and may contribute significantly to the cost of health services for the insurer or healthcare commissioners [5]. These incentives and administrative costs affect the overall cost of health services and the cost varies depending on the payment mechanism.

The thick purple arrow emendating from the middle outputs column is pointing to the intended outcome (reduction of the overall health services cost). The small box that appears in the lower part illustrates efficiency as a criterion used for the analysis of provider payment mechanisms. The use of incentives, cost and efficiency in this study is explicitly defined in the following three subsections.

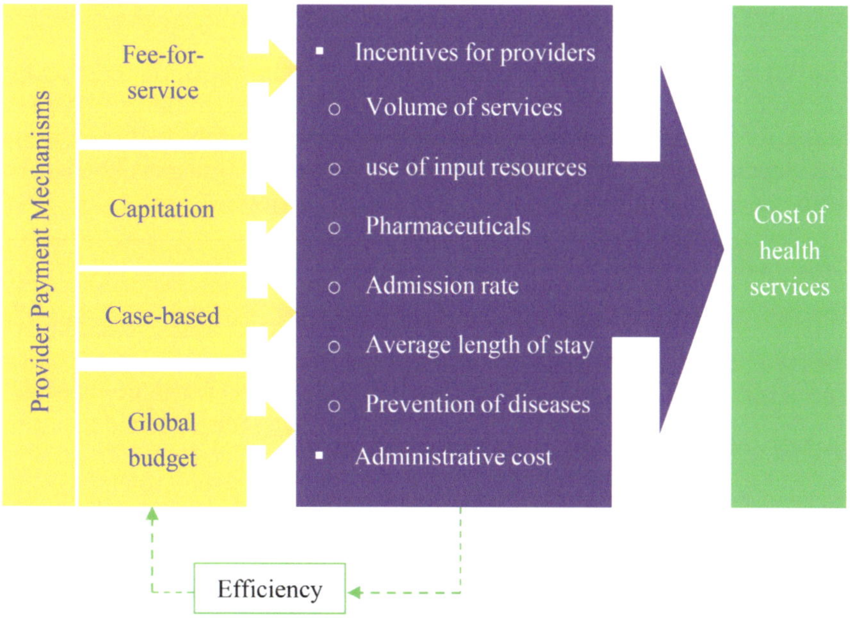

Figure 1.
Conceptual framework for the analysis of provider payment mechanisms.

2.1.1.1 Incentives

Incentives are defined in microeconomics as economic signals that can direct healthcare providers towards self-interested behaviours [1]. These behaviours can lead to beneficial or un-intended effects [6]. For example, one payment mechanism can encourage irrational use of pharmaceuticals as an unintended effect, while another mechanism can promote a reduction in the average length of stay in hospitals as a beneficial effect.

2.1.1.2 Costs

Costs refer to direct cost related to health services covered and reimbursed by health insurance schemes (or other payers) and have two components: (a) direct medical cost such as pharmaceuticals, consultations and laboratory tests and (b) direct non-medical cost such as administrative costs for processing provider claims for reimbursement [7]. These represent the cost from the healthcare system perspective, which this review aims to reduce.

2.1.1.3 Efficiency

Efficiency criterion is used to show the relationship between provider payment mechanisms and their incentives to promote effective and efficient use of resources to produce maximum outputs in health care [1, 4, 8]. By promoting efficiency at the supply side through different payment mechanisms, the overall cost of health services for healthcare systems may be reduced.

2.1.2 Justification and use of the conceptual framework

This conceptual framework represents the key aspects to be analysed in this review, thus keeping the analysis focused. It also helps to articulate the relationships between provider payment mechanisms and their relative incentives and administrative cost, which impacts on the cost of health services.

The framework will be used in Section 3 to discuss the role of the existing FFS payment mechanism in increasing the cost of health services for LMICs. While in Section 4, the framework will be used to guide the critical analysis of the alternative provider payment mechanisms (capitation, case-based and global budget) and assess their potential in reducing the cost of health services.

2.2 Criteria for assessing the feasibility of proposed measures

This has been adapted from [9, 10], and it includes (i) technical feasibility: this will be used in Section 4 to assess the potential of alternative payment mechanisms to control cost and (ii) organisational, financial and cultural feasibility: this will be used in Section 5 to assess the feasibility of implementing the proposed measures in LMIC context.

2.3 Data sources and selection of papers for the review

2.3.1 Data sources

A number of sources of information were used to collect secondary data for this review. These sources are grouped into four categories:

- Electronic databases: web of science, global health and science direct electronic databases.
- Internet search engines: University of Leeds's Library electronic catalogue and Google Scholar were the search engines used to find the full text of selected articles.
- International Organisations' websites: World Bank, WHO and ILO. Research articles and working papers focused on the topic were retrieved from websites of these organisations.
- Other sources of data: books, grey literature and author experiences.

2.3.2 Inclusion and exclusion criteria

Inclusion criteria include: (i) only articles published in English; (ii) articles on health insurance, national health insurance and social health insurance with FFS, capitation, case-based and global budget; (iii) articles from LMIC context and (iv) articles published after 1990 to consider the dynamics in implementing provider payment mechanisms.

Exclusion criteria include: (i) articles focused on health insurance coverage, premiums and benefit packages; (ii) articles discussing other provider payment mechanisms such as per diem, line item budget and pay for performance; (iii) articles focused mainly on developed countries were excluded due to variation from the LMICs context and (iv) articles published before 1990 in order to get the most updated evidence.

2.4 Limitations of the review

The main limitation of this review is the lack of published data from many LMICs for the analysis of country-specific existing provider payment system. However, the author has relied on grey literature including internal reports, conference presentations, other government documents and personal experience. Fortunately, evidence from some LMICs where the widely used FFS payment mechanism was implemented is available in the literature and has been utilised for analysis of the existing provider payment mechanism in Section 3.

The author is also aware that there are other mechanisms for provider payment to tackle the increase in healthcare cost including pay for performance, which may be seen as a limitation. However, this review focuses only on the above-mentioned three alternative payment mechanisms mainly because of the experience of their implementation in LMICs.

In summary, this section described this review as an in-depth study primarily based on secondary data. It described the conceptual framework and its use in this review for analysis for provider payment mechanisms. It described four sources of information used for data collection: electronic databases, search engines, international organisations' websites and other sources of information from LMICs. It highlighted the inclusion and exclusion criteria applied to select relevant papers for the review. The next section analyses existing FFS payment mechanism and its contribution to cost escalation in LMIC context.

3. Analysing the existing fee-for-service provider payment mechanism

Having discussed the conceptual framework for the analysis of provider payment mechanisms and the sources of data used in Section 2, this section analyses the existing FFS payment mechanism and its contribution in increasing the cost of health services for LMICs. There is a continuous escalation in the cost of health services, partly as a result of the implementation of FFS payment for reimbursement of healthcare providers in many LMICs.

3.1 The existing fee-for-service provider payment mechanism in LMICs

FFS is defined as a method for retrospective payment to reimburse healthcare providers for each unit of service provided [11]; for example, the unit of service can be a GP consultation or a laboratory test. Evidence suggests that healthcare systems in many LMICs rely entirely on FFS to reimburse healthcare providers including at primary care, outpatient departments and hospitals.

3.1.1 Fee-for-service incentives to oversupply services and pharmaceuticals

FFS creates strong incentives to provide services with high fee schedules, oversupply of the quantity of services and irrationally increase utilisation of pharmaceuticals; therefore, it leads to cost escalation [6, 12, 13]. Based on the conceptual framework, the following two subsections will analyse the incentives created by FFS to increase the volume of supplied services and induce irrational utilisation of pharmaceuticals as two main contributors for cost escalation in LMICs.

3.1.1.1 Fee-for-service incentives to increase the volume of services

FFS leads to excessive use of services by promoting supplier-induced demand phenomenon since insured patients depend on providers' information on their needs for healthcare [5]. This phenomenon is even higher under circumstances of third-party payers such as insurance-financed services [7]. This is because both providers and patients do not bear the financial risk for the cost of service provided [14]. From the author's experience, this practice can create satisfaction among patients who believe that high quantities and/or expensive treatments mean good quality of health care.

From the author's experience, there is a remarkable perception among insured patients to overuse healthcare services. This moral hazard is another phenomenon associated with increasing demand for free or subsidised service [15]. Such phenomena may continue to increase with the existing FFS reimbursement policy. This has added effect to increase utilisation of services and therefore contributes to cost escalation.

For instance in the National Health Insurance Fund in Sudan, the diagnostic and laboratory services account for 89% of all outpatient visits of which 92% was reported as visits for laboratory tests [16]. This implies significant irrationality in the use of service induced by FFS payment. This relationship is supported by the findings of a systematic review study that was conducted to compare capitation, salary and FFS payment mechanisms. The study revealed that FFS payment results in more primary care visits, specialist visits and more utilisation of diagnostic and curative services compared to capitation and salary payments [12]. Similar findings have been reported in Poland, where the average number of visits for dentists contracted under FFS payment was more than double compared to that provided by salaried dentists [17].

FFS is known for its potential to increase the number of patient visits to primary care, specialised, diagnostic and curative health services [12]. As thus, it contributes to the increased volume of provided services to meet the interest of providers leading to cost escalation.

3.1.1.2 Fee-for-service encourages over utilisation of pharmaceuticals

The cost of pharmaceuticals represents a big proportion of overall healthcare expenditure in LMICs (in some cases reached more 50%). During the past two decades, many interventions were implemented in various LMICs, including enforcement for implementing essential drug lists and increasing awareness among prescribers through rational drug use activities. However, the cost of pharmaceuticals continues to represent a high proportion of overall healthcare expenditure in many LMICs. Evidence from Taiwan showed that 94.3% of hospitals aggressively cut the costs of pharmaceuticals as a response to the shift from FFS to a case-based payment that was implemented by the National Health Insurance Programme in 1995 [18].

From the author's experience, the pharmaceutical industry is also adding pressures on doctors to prescribe new medicines with a higher and sometimes unjustifiable cost. Under the FFS environment, where there are no limits for reimbursing medicine prescriptions, this factor represents one of the major challenges for health insurance schemes to control the cost of pharmaceuticals.

The absence of Standard Treatment Guidelines (STGs) for use of pharmaceuticals in many LMICs (except for few conditions such as malaria and tuberculosis) has worsened the situation and added more incentives for providers to irrationally supply expensive and more quantities of medicines. For example, according to the author, a doctor can prescribe cefixime capsules to treat typhoid fever instead of chloramphenicol capsules as first-line treatment. The former drug could be 10 times more expensive than the later, which significantly contributes to the overall cost of treating typhoid fever cases. The author considers the absence of STGs for pharmaceuticals as one of the major challenges for LMICs to control cost escalation under the current widely used FFS payment system.

Co-payment or cost-sharing may be considered as a way to minimise the effect of FFS on cost escalation. However, evidence from Korea revealed that co-payment alone is not sufficient to tackle the increased volume of health services induced by healthcare providers [5]. Therefore, additional measures might be required to control the rising cost of pharmaceuticals for LMICs.

3.1.2 Administrative cost of fee-for-service

The administrative cost for FFS payment is generally higher compared to other provider payment mechanisms since the insurer is required to process the auditing of detailed provider claims retrospectively based on smaller units [5]. From the author's knowledge, the poor management information system (MIS) has a negative impact on the administrative efficiency to check the accuracy of data submitted by providers. However, FFS has an advantage that the system is easy to design and implement with minimal institutional capacity and training [1].

3.2 Moving away from fee-for-service

As seen up to now, the contribution of FFS in increasing the cost of health services for LMICs was identified. This section will discuss the need for reform from FFS to other methods in order to promote cost containment.

Evidence from LMIC has shown a significant escalation of the cost associated with FFS payment. For example, in Taiwan, the annual per capita health expenditure increased by 15.7% during the period 1980–1994 [19]; and 20% annual cost escalation was reported in Thailand during the period between 1988 and 1997 as result of FFS payment [20].

Due to the unintended effects of FFS, many countries in Asia and Latin America have implemented different reforms to their provider payment systems. For example, Korea and Taiwan implemented reforms from FFS to case-based and global budgeting mixed payment systems [6, 21]; in Argentina, there was significant reform where they moved from FFS to capitation payment [6]; and a report from World Bank suggested that China was advised to move away from FFS in order to control cost escalation in healthcare utilisation [22].

Based on the evidence explored from LMIC on FFS payment, many LMICs may need to consider moving away from FFS to improve efficiency and overcome the problem of cost escalation. The analysis for the alternative payment mechanisms in the next section will help to propose an appropriate reform for each specific context based on the best available evidence.

To summarise this section, the problem of cost escalation of health services for LMICs was demonstrated as partly attributed to the widely used FFS payment mechanism, as one of the main contributing factors. Then the FFS payment mechanism was analysed, and its potential in promoting excessive use of health services, rising cost of pharmaceuticals, and its higher administrative cost, were discussed. Finally, the section concluded with the necessities for LMICs to move away from FFS towards a more appropriate method for reimbursement of healthcare providers in order to tackle cost escalation.

In the next section, capitation, case-based and global budget hospital payment mechanisms will be analysed and the appropriate options for LMICs will be identified.

4. Assessing the alternative provider payment mechanisms

Section 3 discussed the role of the FFS payment mechanism as a contributing factor to cost escalation and suggested that healthcare systems in LMICs need to move away from FFS if cost escalation is to be controlled. This section will analyse three alternative payment mechanisms, capitation, case-based and global budget, and assess their potential to reduce the cost of health services for LMICs. The key issues analysed in this section are those illustrated in the conceptual framework (Section 2), particularly the incentives created by each payment mechanism and the relative administrative cost.

Unlike the retrospective FFS payment, capitation, case-based and global budget payments are prospective mechanisms. The term prospective refers to when the payment rate for a predefined package of health services for the fixed period of time is determined before the treatment takes place [10]. The units of payment are much more aggregated ranging from case treated, with case-based to the health facility, with a global budget [4].

4.1 Capitation payment mechanism

Capitation payment is defined as prospective, fixed payment to healthcare providers in order to care for a defined population for a defined period of time such as a year [11]. The key issue is that reimbursement for providers is not linked to inputs (such as diagnostic tests) or to the volume of service provided. Under capitation payment, providers bear more financial risk for the oversupply of services; therefore, they are more likely to use low inputs in healthcare to retain surplus and make profits [4, 23].

4.1.1 Capitation payment incentives

According to Cashin [24], capitation payment can create incentives for providers for efficiency improvement, the attraction of additional enrollees, an investment in cost-effective health promotion and prevention interventions.

On the other hand, capitation payment can reduce the quality of care, encourages providers not to enrol risky vulnerable patients and results in increased referrals to other providers [25–27]. Jegers et al. [26] suggested that this problem can be solved in the design of capitation payment rates by including risk adjustors (such as age, gender, chronic illness and socio-economic status of enrolled patients). The aim of this risk adjustment is to compensate providers for the higher predicted cost for the care of more costly groups of enrollees such as elderly patients.

Evidence from Thailand has revealed that the introduction of capitation payment in 1990 turned the main contracted providers into risk bearers. They, therefore, became financially responsible for the cost of healthcare for each enrolled patient [28]. This has created incentives to increase the risk pool by expanding population coverage through more enrolment and pass the risk to other subcontracted providers [28].

In the following subsections, three aspects affecting the cost of health services based on the conceptual framework discussed in Section 2 will be analysed. This will focus on incentives to improve efficiency, reducing volume and intensity of supplied service and promoting investment in prevention of diseases.

4.1.1.1 Capitation incentives to improve providers' efficiency

Capitation payment creates strong incentives to promote efficiency in the use of resources [4]. Since providers bear more financial risk for services they provide under capitation payment, they are more likely to control cost by selecting rational and cost-effective services [5]. This is because when providers achieve efficiency gains and spend less than the per capita allocated budget, the difference between revenue and expenditure is maximised, and this surplus is retained by the provider as profit. On the other hand, if a provider runs out of budget, there is no additional payment under the capitation system [24].

Efficiency under a well-designed capitation payment system is promoted by the autonomy and flexibility in the use of resources [1]. This is because the available resources are closely linked to the number of population to be served as well as the health needs of each population [10]. This formula does not only encourage cost minimisation but also improves equity in the distribution of healthcare resources according to the health status of a population [1]. This directs providers to put more emphasis on primary and outpatient care rather than specialised and inpatient services [25].

The degree of incentives created by capitation payment depends on many issues including the health insurance benefit package, the regulations and medical practices existing in the system to prevent risk selection and the healthcare market structure [5]. For example, the availability of other competing providers in the same field encourages efficiency and patient satisfaction. Fortunately, the current health market structure in many LMICs can encourage competition because of the availability of enough numbers of healthcare facilities to ensure competition.

4.1.1.2 Capitation incentives to reduce the volume and intensity of supplied services

Capitation payment can effectively achieve the cost reduction goal by creating incentives for providers to control inpatient admissions and the average length of stay, and review the medical necessity for providing each service [29].

In addition, providers may sacrifice the quality of health services in order to contain costs [10]. Although quality is not the focus of this study, there is a continuous fight between reducing cost and improving quality of health services. Policy makers in LMICs need to make the necessary measures to ensure good quality of care under the expected reform in the provider payment system.

In Thailand, capitation payment was introduced in 1990 with the primary goal to contain the cost of healthcare [10]. As expected, evidence from Thailand has shown that providers responded to capitation incentives by greatly shifting to ambulatory outpatient care and reduced the inpatient services [6, 10]. To cope with this reform, providers undertook certain measures to reduce their cost for managing patients; for example, some hospitals dropped payment for doctor consultations by 30% for Social Security patients compared to regular patients [20].

4.1.1.3 Capitation incentives to invest in health promotion and disease prevention

When capitation payments are contracted for long-term periods with additional bonuses as incentives, providers invest in improving the health status of populations through more cost-effective health services like promotion and prevention interventions [5, 24, 29]. In Nicaragua, for example, capitation payment introduced in 1994 resulted in the adoption of a mixture of services with more emphasis on prevention and primary care than specialised high-level care [25]. This ultimately resulted in a reduction in the overall bill of healthcare for the Social Security Institute in Nicaragua [25].

4.1.2 Administrative cost of capitation payment

This is significantly lower than that of FFS because there are no claims to be processed on the insurer side [5]. Instead, the insurer is only required to audit the number of enrollees per provider to make the payment. However, a well-functioning referral system is required to ensure the cost-effectiveness of treatment at the selected level of care [10].

Administrative costs for managing capitation payment may increase if the health insurance decides to intervene in minimising risk selection by adding risk adjustors such as gender, age or chronic illness of enrolled patients [5, 24]. In such situations, the insurer incurs a more administrative cost for monitoring and tracking patients' enrolment for each provider. Although this can be a negative effect that increases cost, it promotes equity in healthcare and contributes to the overall aim of social health insurance schemes in LMICs.

4.2 Case-based payment mechanism

Case-based is a prospective reimbursement mechanism in which hospitals are paid for each discharged inpatient case, based on a previously defined rate for each group of cases with similar clinical conditions and resource requirement [30]. The International Classification of Diseases (ICD) developed by WHO is widely used to define these groups for the purpose of setting payment rates [1].

4.2.1 Case-based payment incentives

Case-based payment mechanism provides significant incentives for cost reduction [5, 31, 32]. The output-based design of this method has generated major incentives for providers to contain cost per case by minimising the use of resources utilised per case [5], for example, reducing the unnecessary utilisation of diagnostic and imaging services.

Unlike FFS, case-based payment has the potential to create incentives for promoting hospital efficiency and control the cost of healthcare [1, 24, 33]. However, it also encourages contracted hospitals to unnecessarily increase admissions and readmissions, reduce the intensity and quality of care, avoid severe cases and shift patients for outpatient and community care for follow-up [24, 33].

Based on the conceptual framework, the following three subsections will analyse the relevant incentives that contribute to the cost of healthcare under case-based reimbursement.

4.2.1.1 Case-based payment promotes hospital efficiency

Hospital efficiency under cased-based payment is promoted through minimising the inputs used for case management and reducing the average length of stay as intended effects [24, 31, 33]. This is because hospitals are paid a fixed rate for each case regardless of the volume and intensity of service provided.

Case-based payment has been effectively used in many LMICs as a tool to control cost escalation during the past four decades. Stronger incentives to promote efficiency by controlling resources used per case were observed in Korea, Taiwan, Indonesia, China and Kyrgyz Republic [1, 18, 34]. For example, in Korea, the introduction of case-based payment in 1997 resulted in a 30% reduction in the use of antibiotics for inpatient care [21].

In Latin America, case-based payment has also been in existence for the past 30 years, including in Argentina, Brazil and Chile [10]. In Brazil, for example, a mixed case-based and FFS payment system was introduced for reimbursement of both public and private healthcare providers [6]. Although this reform has created incentives for efficiency, evidence has shown that the low reimbursement rates have resulted in negative effects including the deterioration in quality of care and reduced utilisation rates [6, 10].

4.2.1.2 Case-based incentives to increase admission rates

A common problem with case-based payment is that it creates incentives for hospitals to increase admission and readmission rates [33]. However, one of the major advantages associated with case-based payment is the reduction in the average length of stay [24, 35], and it may create incentives for improving quality of care if payment rates are linked to the complexity of cases [10]. For example, the payment rate for complicated normal deliveries is higher than non-complicated ones.

In the Korean reform, the average length of stay has dropped by 3% on average as a response to case-based implementation [21]. The outcome of implemented case-based payment in Kazakhstan during the period 1988–2001 has resulted in a stabilised number of hospital admission rate, a decline in inappropriate admissions, and the average length of stay has dropped by 2 days on average [24].

In Taiwan, evidence has shown that during the first half year after implementation of case-based reform, both the average length of stay and cost per caesarean section admissions dropped significantly [6]. This reform has been confronted with resistance from providers in Taiwan, but the insurer has utilised historical claims data to fairly set the case rates in order to minimise resistance from providers [6, 19]. Consequently, the coping strategies used by hospitals for inpatient admissions in Taiwan as a response to the implementation of case-based payment generally resulted in significant positive outcomes towards cost control [18].

4.2.1.3 Case-based incentives to reduce the intensity of care

Case-based payment has other major disadvantages including incentives to reduce the intensity of healthcare by prematurely discharging admitted patients, up-coding to higher classes in the payment schedule and shifting patterns of care and costs to non-case-based classes where mixed payment systems are used [1, 5]. The behaviour of premature discharge shifts the cost of healthcare from the hospital to the outpatient services and community outreach care, which contributes to increasing the social cost for healthcare. It could also result in high readmission rates [36].

Evidence has shown that up-coding to a higher point practised by providers was not random, but it was systematically favoured by providers and mainly driven by their interest to obtain larger reimbursements [5]; and if the insurer has not taken appropriate measures to reduce this behaviour, the cost of healthcare will increase.

However, Kwon [31] suggested that if the level of care is too high due to the oversupply of services, then the reduction in the intensity of care as a result of implementing case-based payment does not affect patient outcome negatively. Evidence from the Taiwanese experience also supports this point, where irrational use of antibiotics for inpatients was reduced by 30% to cope with case-based payment [18].

4.2.2 Administrative cost of case-based payment

The administrative cost of the case-based payment system primarily depends on the complexity of design for case grouping. The cost of administrating very complex case-based payment is very high for both providers to code cases, and for the insurer to monitor and process provider claims [5]. However, this cost can be lower than FFS in simply designed systems such as those used in Indonesia in the 1990s [5]. In Korea, the relatively high requirement for clinical and managerial information for case classification has been evident [31].

To avoid the higher administrative cost, less complex case-based systems can be designed based on broader categories of case grouping [1]. This approach has also been proposed by Kwon [31], to adopt an incremental implementation of the new case-based system starting with a simpler classification of diseases.

4.3 Global budget hospital payment mechanism

Global budget payment is defined as an aggregate cash sum, fixed in advance, intended to cover the total cost of a service provided, and it is usually set for 1 year ahead [37]. While the unit of payment in capitation payment is per enrollee, in the global budget, the facility is used as a unit of payment based on previous historical spending, the volume of service and hospital bed size, which are brought together in a resource allocation formula [1, 38]. Global budget provides a greater degree of hospital autonomy and increases transparency through the ease of auditing and accountability for allocated budgets and contributes to macro-economic efficiency [38].

Based on the middle purple column of the conceptual framework (Section 2), the following subsections will focus on the analysis of incentives created by global budget payment and the relative administrative cost to run the system.

4.3.1 Global budget payment incentives

Global budget has a positive effect on controlling health insurance cost by creating incentives for hospitals to reduce the volume of services provided and encourages efficient resource utilisation [5]. Depending on the resource allocation formula, global budgeting has both positive and negative effects on the admission rate and the average length of stay in hospital [14].

4.3.1.1 Global budget incentive to reduce the volume of services

With global budget, the volume of healthcare provided is minimised by hospitals due to the shared financial risk [39]. In the short term, the volume of healthcare and use of input resources are minimised and, therefore, can promote hospital efficiency [1, 5]. However, in the long-term period, the degree of incentives brought by this mechanism depends mainly on the resource allocation formula [5] and budget adjustor such as age, sex, morbidity and utilisation rates from previous years [10]. In this regard, policymakers of the health insurer need to keep their attention while using historical data for allocating resources to hospitals, because there are greater chances of repeating existing patterns of resource use. For example, if a non-efficient hospital is receiving global budget based on previous data, without consideration to other adjustors, inefficiency will continuously persist.

Based on the logic discussed above, if other resource allocation adjustors and performance measures are not considered, global budgeting will reward inefficient hospitals (higher spending now to ensure higher budget next year) [38].

4.3.1.2 Effect of global budget on admission rate and the average length of stay

The admission rates are also reduced under global budgeting since contracted hospitals bear some financial risk [4, 5]. When performance measures are introduced in the resource allocation, incentives among hospitals may change as a response to the chosen indicators [38]. For example, in Hungary, the average length of stay increased because global budgets were allocated based on occupancy rates [5].

The major disadvantages of global budget payment are that it is not reflective of the actual activities carried out by the hospital, but rather it is based on the hospital bed capacity [38]. Unfortunately, complicated cases are also treated with the same level of funding, which may lead to the referral of severe cases [10, 38]. This can be minimised by introducing more complex resource allocation formula to reflect the severity of cases [10].

4.3.2 Administrative cost of global budget

The administrative cost of the global budget is generally lower compared to other payment methods [5]. This cost is mainly brought by the resource allocation formula and there are no bills to prepare and no claim audits [1]. But, this cost may increase when using more complex resource allocation formulas such as risk-adjusted or utilisation projection components in the formula [5, 38].

The administrative cost is also possible to increase by introducing better monitoring of performance measures such as result-based assessment and evaluation for hospitals contracted under a global budget [38, 40].

4.4 Which payment mechanism is the best for LMICs?

Policy makers in LMICs need to understand that all provider payment mechanisms have advantages and disadvantages and there is no perfect method. Langenbrunner [41] stated that “the whole point of provider payment systems is to change behaviour”: that is, to change the way healthcare providers operate in response to different incentives discussed in this study under each method while achieving the policy objective of cost containment.

Mixed payment systems are widely used in different countries in Asia and Latin America: for example, (FFS, case-based and capitation) in Kyrgyzstan and Argentina, and (FFS and case-based) in Chile and Brazil [10]. The mixed system is adopted for practical reasons to counter the adverse incentives of using pure payment mechanisms [5]. For example, hospitals can be reimbursed on case-based, while primary care centres can be paid on a capitation basis. Mixed systems can even be used for one provider. This has been successful in Thailand where hospitals are reimbursed on a global budget to cover fixed costs and partly on case-based to cover variable costs for emergency cases [42].

According to Wouters [10], three main issues need to be considered when preparing for a payment system reform: (i) the potential of the payment mechanism to control cost; (ii) the supporting system requirement for implementing the new payment system and (iii) the expected effect on quality of care. Since quality of care is out of the scope of this review, only the first two elements (i and ii) are summarised in the following two subsections.

4.4.1 The potential of alternative payment mechanisms to control cost

Based on the analysis for provider payment mechanisms, the discussion above summarised the findings of key incentives and administrative costs for the three alternative payment mechanisms. The summary of findings from the analysis of the existing FFS payment is presented for comparison purposes (**Table 1**).

As you can see in **Table 1**, each of the alternative payment mechanisms creates both positive and negative incentives and all of them are technically feasible to reduce healthcare costs. However, case-based has higher administrative cost compared to capitation and global budget. In terms of organisational feasibility, the case-based method also requires a higher institutional capacity to run the system. Therefore, capitation and global budget may be the most viable options for LMICs.

4.4.2 Supporting system requirements for implementation

The success of provider payment mechanisms cannot be achieved as stand-alone interventions; other supporting measures are equally important including legal, financial, referral, quality assurance and MIS [10]. For example, capitation payment requires a very well-developed referral system to operate effectively, while case-based payment relies on a well-designed and functioning information system to ensure accurate coding and keeping clinical records for each case managed. **Figure 2** illustrates the relative level of complexity for supporting system requirements for implementing provider payment mechanisms.

To summarise this section, the three alternative provider payment mechanisms were analysed: capitation, case-based and global budget. The conceptual

Payment mechanism	Incentives	Administrative cost
Capitation	+ Improves provider efficiency + Reduces volume and intensity of service + Invests in health promotion and disease prevention – Selection of healthier enrollees	Low
Case-based	+ Improves hospital efficiency + Reduces the volume of inputs – Increases admission and readmission rates – Reduces the intensity of care	High
Global budget	– Reduces the volume of supplied services ± Increases or decreases admission rate and averages length of stay depending on resource allocation formula and performance measures – May reward inefficient hospitals	Low
Fee-for-service	– Does not promote provider efficiency – Increases volume of supplied service – Overutilization of pharmaceuticals + Improves access to healthcare	High

Key: +, positive incentives; –negative incentives.

Table 1.
Findings from analysis for provider payment mechanisms.

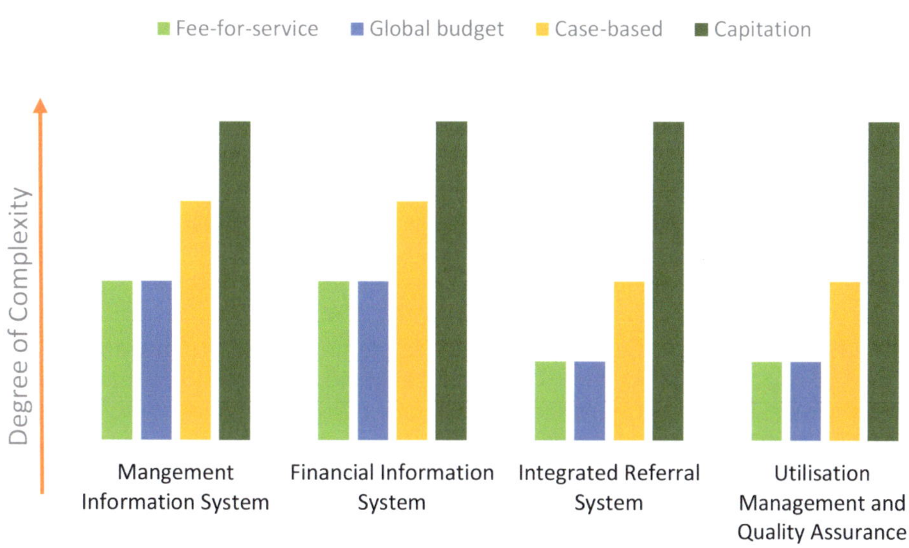

Figure 2.
Supporting system requirements. Source: adapted from [10].

framework was used in the analysis and assessed the positive and negative incentives created by each payment mechanism. The relative administrative cost to run each of these mechanisms and their potential in controlling the cost of health services were also analysed. The relative requirements for supporting systems to run each of the alternative provider payment mechanisms were also identified and compared.

The next section will present the conclusions of this study and potential measures for provider payment reform in LMICs.

5. Conclusions

5.1 General conclusions

This chapter discussed the problem of cost escalation for providing healthcare in LMICs and analysed the existing FFS payment method for reimbursement of healthcare providers as the main contributor to this problem.

FFS payment significantly contributes to cost escalation by creating incentives for providers to unnecessarily increase the volume of supplied health services and irrationally increase the utilisation of pharmaceuticals. Moreover, the administrative cost of FFS is relatively high compared to capitation and global budget payment mechanisms. Evidence from LMIC in Asia and Latin America revealed a number of reforms during the past four decades where they moved away from FFS to prospective payment mechanisms to promote cost containment.

Fortunately, the analysis of findings from the assessment of the alternative provider payment mechanisms has demonstrated the potential of these methods in controlling cost and promoting efficiency. Capitation payment and global budget hospital payment mechanisms may be the two viable alternative options for implementation in LMICs.

Both capitation and global budget payment mechanisms create strong incentives for providers to reduce the volume of supplied health services and their administrative cost is low compared to the existing FFS payment method. Capitation payment has the potential to promote provider efficiency, while global budgeting may negatively reward inefficient hospitals if risk adjustors (such as gender and age) are not applied in the resource allocation formula.

Interestingly, capitation payment encourages healthcare providers to invest in health promotion and disease prevention activities to improve the health status of enrolled populations, but it can also discriminate against enrolling risky vulnerable and costly groups and select healthier enrollees.

Mixed provider payment systems can be used to absorb the adverse effects of using a pure payment mechanism and also for practical reasons in implementation. The success of implementing capitation and global budget payment mechanisms in LMICs requires other supporting systems with different degrees of complexity. Therefore, LMICs need to invest in strengthening both the financial information system and MIS. In addition, the utilisation management and quality assurance systems need to be introduced in the contractual requirements where separate payers such as health insurance schemes exist.

5.2 Potential measures for provider payment reform in LMICs

Based on the existing evidence and analysis provided in this chapter, a set of technically feasible potential measures is proposed for LMICs. The measures are summarised in two groups: short-term and long-term measures with a discussion of the feasibility (organisational, financial and cultural) for implementing each of these measures in LMIC context.

5.2.1 Short-term measures

- Adopt a policy reform for gradually shifting away from FFS towards the implementation of capitation and global budget provider payment mechanisms for reimbursement of healthcare providers.

- Fair setting of reimbursement rates in the new payment system is required to avoid resistance from healthcare providers that may arise as a response to the proposed reform.

- Design of a mixed provider payment system with the following directions:

    - Capitation payment for reimbursement to primary care facilities.

    - Global budget payment for smaller and district hospitals.

    - FFS payment may remain as a method for reimbursement to outpatient departments and specialised healthcare, where appropriate.

- Make the necessary measures to keep the quality of healthcare at an acceptable level under the newly designed provider payment system as part of reform packages.

- Design and implementation of payment system reform are lengthy and detailed processes and need a legal framework for implementation (legislation).

- Recruit technical support from World Bank, WHO or other specialised institutions for designing the new provider payment system, which should include setting the payment rates, resource allocation formula, billing system and improving the institutional capacity to run the new system. Technical support can be obtained through multilateral or bilateral development of cooperation projects.

- Strengthen the supporting systems to the relative degree of requirements to run the new provider payment system. These include the financial information system, MIS, integrated referral system and utilisation management and quality assurance system.

- A large amount of financial investment, as well as training for human resources to administer the new system, is required.

5.2.2 Long-term measures

- Evaluate the newly introduced provider payment system to assess its effectiveness in controlling the cost of health services and make periodical adjustments for payment rates based on data generated from the previous experience. A well-functioning MIS and reasonable financial budget are required to conduct this evaluation.

- Expand capitation payment for reimbursement of health services provided at the primary care level. All supporting systems are required to be functioning to a higher degree of complexity.

- Expand global budget payment for reimbursement of contracted hospitals. A well-functioning MIS is required to apply risk adjustors (such as age and sex) in the resource allocation formula. Financial and human resources need to be mobilised for monitoring and evaluation of performance measures for participating hospitals.

Acknowledgements

The author acknowledges that an early version of this report has been submitted in partial fulfilment of the requirements for the award of Master of Public Health (International) at Nuffield Centre for International Health and Development, University of Leeds, UK.

Author details

Abualbishr Alshreef
School of Health and Related Research, University of Sheffield, Sheffield, UK

*Address all correspondence to: a.o.alshreef@sheffield.ac.uk

References

[1] Langenbrunner JC, Cashin C, O'Dougherty S. Designing and Implementing Health Care Provider Payment Systems: How-to Manuals. Washington, DC: World Bank; 2009

[2] WHO. World Health Report, Health Systems Financing: The Path to Universal Coverage. Geneva: World Health Organization; 2010. pp. 87-97

[3] Alshreef A et al. Cost-effectiveness of docetaxel and paclitaxel for adjuvant treatment of early breast cancer: Adaptation of a model-based economic evaluation from the United Kingdom to South Africa. Value in Health Regional Issues. 2019;**19**:65-74

[4] Maceira D. Provider payment mechanisms in health care: Incetives, outcomes, and organizational impact in developing countries. In: Major Applied Research 2, Working Paper 2. Partnership for Health Reform Project. Bethesda, MD: Abt Associates Inc; 1998

[5] Barnum H, Kutzin J, Saxenian H. Incentives and provider payment methods. International Journal of Health Planning and Management. 1995;**10**:23-45

[6] Bitran R, Yip WC. A review of health care provider payment reform in seleced countriesd in Asia and Latin America. In: Major Applied Research 2, Working Paper 1. Partnership for Health Reform Project. Bethesda, MD: Abt Associates Inc; 1998

[7] Wonderling D, Gruen R, Black N. Introduction to Health Economics. Glasgow: Bell & Bain Ltd; 2005

[8] McGlynn EA. Identifying, Categorizing, and Evaluating Health Care Efficiency Measures. In: The Southern California Evidence-based Practice Center. Rockville, MD: RAND Corporation; 2008

[9] Wally J, Wright J. Public Health an Action Guide to Improving Health. 2nd ed. Oxford: Oxford University Press; 2010

[10] Wouters A. Alternative provider payment methods: Incentives for improving health care delivery. In: Terrell N, Moll L, Laughrin A, editors. Primer for Policymakers Series. Partnerships for Health Reform. Bethesda, MD: Abt Associates Inc; 1998

[11] Waters HR, Hussey P. Pricing health services for purchasers—A review of methods and experiences. Health Policy. 2004;**70**:175-184

[12] Gosden T, et al. Capitation, Salary, Fee-For-Service and Mixed Systems of Payment: Effect on the Behaviour of Primary Care Physicians (Review). The Cochrance Library; 2009

[13] Cashin C. Fee-For-Service Payment Systems, in Strategic Purchasing for Social Protection: A Short Course for Capacity Development. Bangkok: Centre for Health Economics, Chulalongkorn University; 2009

[14] Preker AS, Langenbrunner JC. Spending Wisely: Buying Health Services for the Poor. Washington, DC: World Bank; 2005

[15] Folland S, Goodman AC, Stano M. The Economics of Health and Health Care. 3rd ed. New Jersey: Printice Hall Inc; 2001

[16] MCoAS, Sudan. National Health Insurance Assessment Study. Khartoum: Muhanna and Co. Actuarial Services; 2007. pp. 1-27

[17] Domagala A et al. Public Service Reforms and Their Impact on Health Sector Personnel in Poland. Krakow: World Health Organization and International Labour Organization; 1999

[18] Huang CC et al. Effectiveness of coping strategies used by hospitals in response to implementation of case-based payment system by ther National Health Insurance Programme. Journal of the Formosan Medical Association. 2005;**104**(7):468-475

[19] Chiang T-l. Taiwan's 1995 health care reform. Health Policy. 1997;**39**(3):225-239

[20] Mills A et al. The response of providers to capitation payment: A case-study from Thailand. Health Policy. 2000;**51**:163-180

[21] Kwon S. Payment system reform for health care providers in Korea. Health Policy and Planning. 2003;**18**(1):84-92

[22] Yip W, Eggleston K. Provider payment reform in China: The case of hospital reimbursement in Hainan Province. Health Economics. 2001;**10**:325-339

[23] Robinson J, Cassalino L. Vertical integration and organizational networks in health care. Health Affairs. 1996;**15**(1):7-22

[24] Cashin C et al. The Design and Implementation of Per Capita Payment Systems in the Context of Primary Health Care-Centered Health System Development in Low- and Midle-Income Countries. Bethesda, MD: Abt Associates, Inc; 2007

[25] Ubilla G, Espinosa C, Bitran R. The use of capitation payment by the social security institute and previsional medical enterprises in Nicaragua. In: Major Applied Research 2, Working Paper 3. Partnership for Health Reform. Bethesda, MD: Abt Associates, Inc.; 2000

[26] Jegers M et al. A typology for provider payment systems in health care. Health Policy. 2002;**60**:255-273

[27] Robinson J. Payment mechanisms, non-price incentives, and organizational innovation in health care. Inquiry. 1993;**30**:228-333

[28] Yip WC et al. Impact of capitation payment: The social security scheme of Thailand. In: Major Applied Research 2, Working Paper 4. Partnerships for Health Reform Project. Bethesda, MD: Abt Associates Inc; 2001

[29] Keckley PH, Underwood HR, Frink B. Episode-Based Payment: Perspectives for Consideration. Washington, DC: Deloitte Center for Health Solutions; 2009

[30] Telyukov A. Prospective case-based payment for hospitals: A guide with illustrations from Latin America. In: Health Sector Reform Initiative. Bethesda, MD: Abt Associates Inc; 2001

[31] Kwon S. Case-based payment systems for health care providers. In: Strategic Purchasing for Social Protection: A Short Course for Capacity Development. Bangkok: Centre for Health Economics, Chulalongkorn University; 2009

[32] Miller HD. From volume to value: Better ways to pay for health care. Health Affairs. 2009;**28**(5):1418-1428

[33] World Bank. Health Provider Payment Reforms in China: What International Experience Tells Us, in Working Paper No. 58414. Washington, DC: World Bank; 2010

[34] Wagstaff A. Health systems in East Asia: What can developing countries learn from Japan and the Asian tigers? Health Economics. 2007;**16**:441-456

[35] World Bank. Healthy Development: The World Bank Strategy for Health, Nutrition and Population Results. Washington, DC: World Bank; 2007

[36] Cashin C et al. Case-based Hospital Payment Systems: A Step-By-Step Guide for Implementation in Low- and Middle-Income Countries. Washington, DC: United States Agency for International Development; 2005

[37] Oxley H, MacFarlan M. Health care reform: Controlling spending and increasing efficiency. In: OECD Economic Studies No. 24. Paris: Organization for Economic Co-operation and Development; 1995

[38] Aljunid SM. Provider payment mechanism: Global budget. In: Strategic Purchasing for Social Protection: A Short Course for Capacity Building. Bangkok: Centre for Health Economics, Chulalongkorn University; 2009

[39] Dredge R. Hospital Global Budgeting, in Health, Nutrition and Population (HNP) Discussion Paper. Washington, DC: World Bank; 2004

[40] Munkhtsetseg AB. Global budget experience in Mongolia. In: Strategic Purchasing for Social Protection: A Short Course for Capacity Building. Bangkok: Centre of Health Economics, Chulalongkorn University; 2009

[41] Langenbrunner JC. Provider payment: Which one? How do you implement. In: Strategic Purchasing for Social Protection: A Course for Capacity Building. Bangkok: Centre for Health Economics, Chulalongkorn University; 2009

[42] Sriratanaban J. Health care purchasing and provider responses in Thailand. In: Strategic Purchasing for Social Protection: A Course for Capacity Building. Bangkok: Centre for Health Economics, Chulalongkorn University; 2009

Chapter 3

Universal Health Coverage, Long-Term Care, and Funding in an Aging Era

Aida Isabel Tavares and Pedro Lopes Ferreira

Abstract

Universal health coverage has been gaining a wider attention since the beginning of the 2000s, and it has become an ideological reference for health systems across the world. Funding universal health coverage has been a major challenge faced by governments. Not only funding has to be efficient to guarantee people's access to health services when they are needed, but also it has to ensure equity across people in the country. Aging implies a new constraint to funding as more people contribute less to the collection of financial revenues and more people are in need of healthcare, due to morbidity and end-of-life needs. This chapter aims to present the concept of universal health coverage and LTC and also to discuss how it may be financed under the current scenario of demographic aging and increasing demand for long-term care.

Keywords: universal health coverage, long-term care, funding, aging

1. Introduction

Universal health coverage (UHC) has been gaining a wider attention since the beginning of the 2000s, and it has become an ideological reference for health systems across the world. UHC stands for ensuring that health services, needed by people, are of sufficient quality, and that people may access them without exposing themselves to financial hardship.

The historical background of UHC goes back to the period immediately after World War II. In 1948, WHO's constitution considered health as a human right; in 1978, the Alma Ata declaration sustained the importance of primary healthcare to grant "Health for All"; in 2005, members of WHO signed a resolution aiming at the implementation of universal coverage [1]; recently, in 2018, in the Declaration of Astana governments recommitted to the importance of primary healthcare as a major pillar of UHC. Additionally, the UN has set UHC as a target for Sustainable Development Goal (SDG 3.8 [2]) to be achieved by 2030 [3].

Funding UHC has been one of the major challenges faced by governments. Not only funding has to be efficient to guarantee people's access to health services when they are needed but it also has to ensure equity across people in the country.

Today governments have to deal with the new reality of aging societies. This demographic phenomenon is taking place all over the world, although some countries are aging more rapidly than others. For instance, in EU, it is expected that within five decades, the number of elderly aged over 80 will triple and there be only two active people (15–64 y.o.[1]) for each older person (+65 y.o.) [4].

Aging implies a new constraint to funding as more people contribute less to the collection of financial revenues and more people are in need of healthcare, due to morbidity and end-of-life needs.

In this chapter, we aim to present the concept of universal health coverage and LTC and also to discuss how it may be financed under the present scenario of demographic aging and increasing demand for long-term care.

2. Universal health coverage and aging

Universal healthcare coverage is the natural evolution of health systems since the World War II. UHC may be described as a general coverage framework where people receive health services needed with quality, without suffering financial hardship [5]. So, the two main objectives may be listed. First, all people should have access to a package of services in wide range of healthcare spectrum, including treatment, promotion, prevention, rehabilitation, long-term care, and palliative care. This objective guarantees that healthcare services may be available to everybody, with quality when they are needed. Therefore, quality and equity are core to this objective.

The second objective ensures that people do not get bankruptcy because of health-care expenditures. The best way to prevent this financial hardship on people is by compulsory prepayment to a fund. The payments done by people are according to their ability to pay, which implies that there are always some people in the population who need to be subsidized because they are poor or cannot contribute to the fund.

UHC requires efficient management and fairness-sustainability trade-offs because UHC does not mean unlimited resources nor services provided. The general long-lasting aim of UHC is to expand coverage on a three- dimensional cube (**Figure 1**): breadth, depth, and height. Breadth of coverage measures the

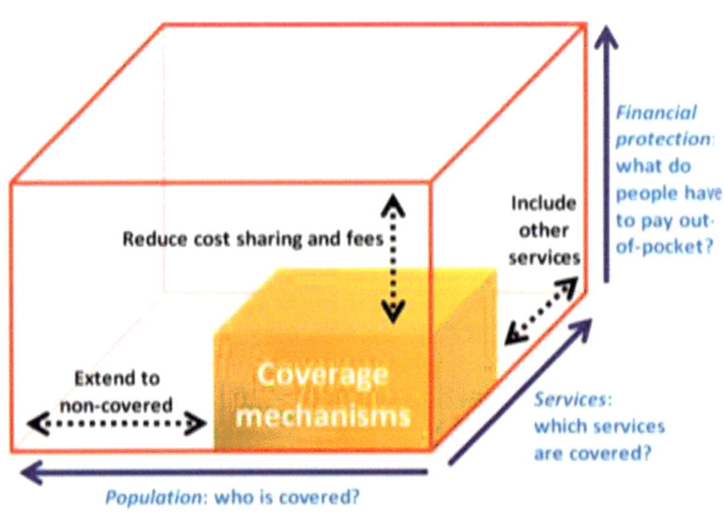

Figure 1.
UHC cube. Source: Based on WHO [6].

[1] y. o.—years old.

proportion of people who are covered or entitled; depth reflects the healthcare services that are included in the package of UHC; and finally, height shows the proportion of costs that are shared between people and the health system.

3. Aging effect

Nowadays aging is a major demographic phenomenon taking placing. People are getting older, and so there is change in the age distribution pictures from a pyramidal shape to inverted pyramidal shape. The fast growing percentage of elderly in the population is expected to take place in the next decades, as shown in **Figure 2,** which displays the projected evolution of older age groups for Europe.

There are three trends that may explain the current aging phenomenon [8]. They include (i) the increased longevity of people as people they live longer, (ii) the declined fertility as women have less children, and (iii) the aging of "baby boom" generations.

This demographic scenario raises the concern of how living longer is related to people's health, in particular, in later stages in life. In fact, the relationship between aging and health has been described from three different perspectives:

i. a compression of morbidity, proposed by Fries [9], where morbidity is condensed in the last part of the life cycle;

ii. an expansion of morbidity, proposed by Gruenber [10] and Kramer [11], where the increased life years are unhealthy and spent with morbidity; and

iii. a dynamic equilibrium, proposed by Manton [12], which is something in between the two previous proposals, meaning that, there is a constant proportion of healthy life in the overall life cycle of people. According to this proposal, the gains obtained of life span without disability are balanced by losses in healthy life span. The dynamic equilibrium may also be described by the balance between the decreasing/constant proportion of life span with serious illness or disability, and the increasing proportion of life span with moderate disability or illness severity.

Depending on the country or the region, these three perspectives may be found. However, in all of them, the increasing need of long-term care (LCT) is inevitable. What may differ across each of them is the kind of LCT needed and provided.

LTC may be defined as the range of services and assistance for people who, as a result of mental and/or physical frailty and/or disability over an extended period of

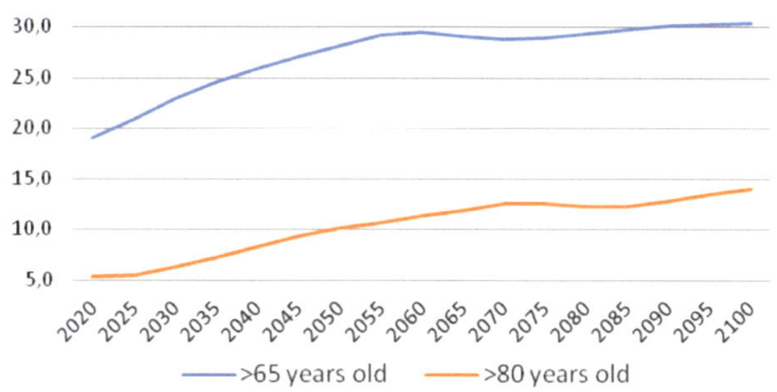

Figure 2.
Projections of percentage of age group in population in Europe. Source: Based on UN data [7]—Based on medium variant projections of age groups for Europe.

time, depend on help with daily living activities and/or are in need of some permanent nursing care" [4]. The living activities for which people may need help include both activities of daily living (ADL) and instrumental activities of daily living (IADL). The ADL include basic self-care tasks such as healthcare and personal care (e.g., help with hygiene) and also household help (e.g., shopping). IADL include activities related to independent living and include preparing meals, managing money, shopping for groceries or personal items, performing light or heavy housework, doing laundry, and using a telephone.

Long-term care is often under looked in the package of UHC, even though its provision has been increasing in several countries, in particular, in Northern Europe. The provision of LTC can take different forms: health or social nature, cash or in-kind benefits, and institutional/formal or home/informal care.

The variability of long-term care systems across countries is so large that comparisons are difficult to perform. For instance, when comparing the long-term care expenditures (both social and health) as a share of current health expenditures across EU countries, it becomes clear that all LTC systems tend to be different (**Figure 3**).

Comparing different forms of LTC provided across countries becomes even harder as shown in **Figure 4**, when comparing expenditures in LTC per capita and the structure of expenditures in type of LTC.

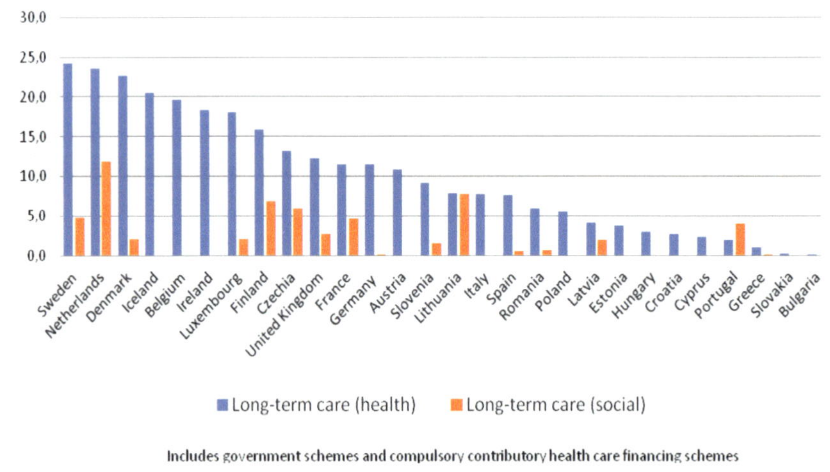

Figure 3.
Share of total current health expenditure (%CHE), 2016. Source: Based on Eurostat data [13].

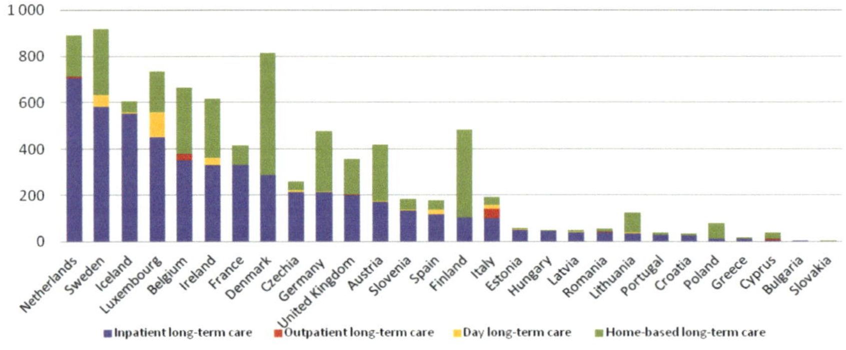

Figure 4.
Expenditures on different types of long-term care, 2016. Note: Includes government schemes and compulsory contributory health-care financing schemes; monetary unit: Purchasing power standard (PPS) per inhabitant. Source: Based on Eurostat data [13].

To overcome comparisons across countries, OECD [14] has proposed one classification of LTC systems. Two criteria are used to classify LTC coverage: one is the depth of the benefits and the other is the organization.

The depth of the benefits measures the scope of the entitlement of the LTC benefits, i.e., either universal or means-tested; the organization criterion assesses how the LCT is covered, either by a single system or by a multiple benefits, services, and programs.

Based on these two criteria, three groups of countries are identified. The first group includes countries with a universal coverage based on a single program (e.g., Nordic countries, Belgium, and Japan). This system may be separate from the health system, or be part it, and LTC is provided to everyone eligible. This does not mean free provision because there may be means of payment such as co-payments or user charges subject to income thresholds.

The second group considers mixed systems (e.g., Italy, Czech Republic, Ireland, Australia, France, Greece, Spain, and Switzerland), meaning a mixture of universal with means-tested LTC programs and benefits. In these countries, there is no single LTC system but rather multiple benefits and entitlements.

Finally, the third group includes countries with means-tested safety net schemes (e.g., USA). Under this type of LTC coverage organization, income and/or assets are used to assess the eligibility to publicly funded care. People with means lower than some established threshold are entitled to receive such coverage.

The allocation of LTC benefits varies across countries, and all countries end up facing the same trade-off between fair protection and fiscal sustainability. The allocation of resources to LTC usually does not provide full costs of LTC to all older people. Benefits are to be distributed according to the three vectors of UHC: eligibility or entitlement rules (breadth), depth of services covered, and the height of cost sharing.

4. UHC, funding, and LTC

Health systems are expected to perform several functions, and funding is one of them. This function financially supports three aims of any health system: improving population health, responding to people expectations, and providing financial protection against the costs of ill health, including health decline due to age [15].

Funding health systems aims to "provide people with access to needed health services, including prevention, promotion, treatment, and rehabilitation, of sufficient quality to be effective and to ensure that the use of those services do not expose people to financial hardship" [15]. According to this definition, there are three roles that funding has to perform: (i) collecting funds, (ii) pooling funds and risk, and (iii) purchasing healthcare services.

Collecting funds means raising revenues, using several sources and contribution mechanisms; pooling funds and risk translates the arrangements to gather the prepaid funds and diversify the individual risk across the pool of participants; purchasing healthcare services comprises the way that the funds are transferred to providers, either by provider payment mechanisms (PPM) or by institutional structure of purchasers [16].

A more in-depth explanation is next presented for each of these roles of funding.

4.1 Collecting funds

Today, it is widely accepted that the best way to fund healthcare systems is based on prepaid mechanism gathered from a large pool of contributing individuals. Funding mechanisms include the voluntary and the mandatory mechanisms (and some low- and medium-income countries (LMIC) may also find external sources of financing obtained from international donors).

Voluntary financing mechanisms account for the out-of-pocket payments and voluntary insurance. Out-of-pocket payments are the most regressive form of funding the health system, and they may contribute to catastrophic expenditures and poverty. Voluntary insurance may be a secondary layer of health insurance but it is inequitable as it does not extend to all people.

Mandatory funding mechanisms are the most efficient mechanism to guarantee a prepaid healthcare expenditure and to finance UHC. There are, however, two basic forms of these mechanisms: social insurance and taxation, each rooted in its historical proponent. The former funding system was proposed by Otto von Bismark, who implemented the sickness funds system financed by payroll taxes in 1883, in Germany. The later funding proposal was given by William Beveridge, who suggested the national health system financed by taxes in 1948, in UK.

These two approaches to finance health systems, either social insurance or tax based, are also the same financing mechanism of long-term healthcare. While the advantages of the tax-based system are the broader base of funding and greater flexibility and adaptability in providing benefits, the social insurance-based system ensures higher transparency and predictable revenues. On the other hand, the tax-based system has no link between the revenues and the provided benefits while the social insurance-based system is inflexible in the benefits awarded and ends up requiring public budget contribution for those who are not able to pay the for the social insurance contribution [17].

The large majority of health systems nowadays is mainly or partially financed by taxes, either because the major financing source is taxes or because insurance funds do not cover the whole population and so complementary financial source is needed.

Low- and middle-income countries with high unequal income distribution face a taxing challenge: to tax the wealthy and powerful country elites to finance in an equitable way the health system of the country. Because in most cases these elites are also the political and governing ones, it ends up that equitable collecting funds for the health system do not occur.

User fees are one source of funding which raise some controversy. While some argue that user fees reduce utilization by poorer people, others consider that user fees cannot be ignored as an important funding source in some countries. In particular, in countries where resources are limited and institutions are weak, as happens in several LMIC. It is argued that if there is a well-designed user's fee policy, which includes waiver mechanisms and compensating procedures to providers, and as long as those public fees are lower than private fees, then user fees may be an efficient and less inequitable source of funding.

Funding LTC either by taxes or by social contribution may not be enough to accommodate all the people in need of care. So other funding alternatives, which may complement taxes or social contributions, are required to be collected.

Wouterse and Smid [18] have proposed four LTC funding mechanisms: (i) pay-as-you-go system, (ii) collective saving funds, (iii) pensioner tax, and (iv) cohort-specific savings. The differences across these alternatives are the distribution of costs along time and across age groups.

i. The pay-as-you-go system is described as a financing system where contributions come from actual workers to pay the current retirement benefits. So the additional spending available for LTC in some year is matched by the additional premium payments collected in that year.

ii. The second funding mechanism is saving fund which is created by the contribution of people. Collective saving funds are a form of pooled funds which aim to generate a steady level of income without threatening the initial value. This idea is basically creating a pre-funding mechanism to be used in the future [19]. Pre-funding may be full or partial. By partial it is meant that LTC contributions are expected to cover only part of the LTC costs of the individual. This partial contribution seems to ensure some intergenerational fairness because the younger generation does not assume the complete burden of LTC costs of an older generation.

iii. The third proposal is the pensioner tax which is a specific tax on pension incomes. This is a premium rate levied on pension income and it provides an increasing source of LTC funding as the group of pensioners is increasing. This works like tax broadening strategy for an intra-generational pooling of funds.

iv. Finally, the idea supporting the cohort-specific savings is that each birth cohort funds its own additional LTC expenditures. This is like tying pre-funding to specific age-related costs as suggested by OECD [19].

4.2 Pooling funds and risk

Pooling funds are a key factor in well-functioning healthcare systems aiming to UHC. Accumulating and managing financial resources from a large pool of individuals ensures that the individual risk of paying for healthcare expenditures is in fact dispersed by all the individuals in the pool. The channel through which such dispersion happens is called cross-subsidization. This takes place by having higher income people paying for lower income people, lower risk people paying for higher illness-risk people, and active people paying for inactive people, such as children and elderly. The second advantage of large pools is the potential to obtain economies of scale and market power. Large funding pools work more efficiently with less administrative costs and with lower negotiated prices.

Countries with fragmented insurance system do not have pools of individuals large enough to ensure that an individual unpredictable financial risk becomes predicted and distributed among all the individuals contributing to the insurance funding pool. This is the case in several LMIC where there may coexist different health insurance. These multiple insurance pools result in increasing administrative costs, individual's selection risk, and individual's segmentation according to income and wealth.

However, the fragmentation of the funding pools is not bad *per se*. Countries may choose to have one pool organized under a single organization or allow the co-existence of several insurances (or pools), which may (or not) compete among themselves. The government decision about the organization and the structure of the pool of individuals has to guarantee that it is equitable and there is no risk selection. So the two necessary conditions to finance a UHC are "compulsion" of a contributions and "subsidization" across individuals, as explained by Fuchs [20]. How these conditions are met depends on the government choice. Pooling against LTC risk is a basic social concern since potentially all citizens are in risk of needing LTC and the poorer ones are at risk of financial hardship.

In aging societies such as in Europe, the group of elderly who are at risk of becoming frail and developing multi-morbidity conditions is large and increasing. So, the risk of being in need of LTC is rising and it requires large pool of funding in order to disperse this risk by all contributors.

4.3 Purchasing healthcare services

Purchasing healthcare services comprises three areas of concern. The first one addresses the decision of which services are included in the package of UHC and which services are to be bought; the second concern is the choice of providers; and the third concern relates on the form to purchasing and provision the healthcare services.

The decision on which services are included is not identical across countries. High-income countries may include services which in LMIC may not be in the UHC package because of strong funding restrictions. These countries may be more interested in including services more suitable for their reality such as malaria-related services, HIV antiretroviral therapy, diphtheria-tetanus-pertussis vaccine, or they may be more interested in improving the quality of the services already provided [21].

Considering that the provided care must be fair and efficient, the decision on the services included in a LTC package may be difficult to decide. OECD [14] has proposed the idea of targeted universalism of LTC, that is, the target of care covered is where the need is highest. This idea grounded on the fact that universal LTC may not be attainable for all, but it should be for those in greatest need [22].

The choice of providers may be passive by just assigning a predetermined budget or paying bills or it may be done strategically, meaning that it is a process that aims to maximize performance [15]. Concerning this choice of providers in LTC care, it is diverse, including health or social sector and from institutional/formal care or home/informal care. Informal care may be funded by public subsidization since this form of care has been accepted as cost-effectiveness [23].

The decision concerning the form of purchasing is highly dominated by the choice of the provider payment mechanisms (PPM) and contractual arrangements (discussed in more detail in Chapter 3 of this book). This choice is fundamental to ensure efficiency and transparency of the system. Provider payment mechanisms have a particular role in providing the correct incentives to providers to guarantee access, quality, and efficiency. The PPM comprises several possible arrangements such as global budget, fee for service, capitation, *per diem*, case based, and pay-for-performance [24].

The organization of the purchasers in the health system depends on the competition established among them. There are different forms of organization of the providers purchasing market as described by Kutzin [16]. The simplest form is the single payer system, where there is only one national institution which is responsible for the payments to providers (e.g., in Japan). When there are multiple payers, meaning multiples insurers, there is a distinction between the case when the population covered is in one area, or in different geographical areas. When it covers different geographical areas, more than one regional body is responsible for purchasing and it is a subset of the simple payer system (e.g., in Canada). If the population covered is in the same geographical area, then there may be, or not, competition for the people covered by the insurers. In this way, there are multiple noncompeting insurers (e.g., in France) or there are multiple competing insurers (e.g., in Germany) [16].

5. Classification of LTC systems in the European Union

Universal long-term healthcare is a difficult concept to achieve and to compare internationally. Several difficulties arise related to the decisions over the three dimensions of UHC: (i) eligibility, (ii) package of services, and (iii) cost sharing.

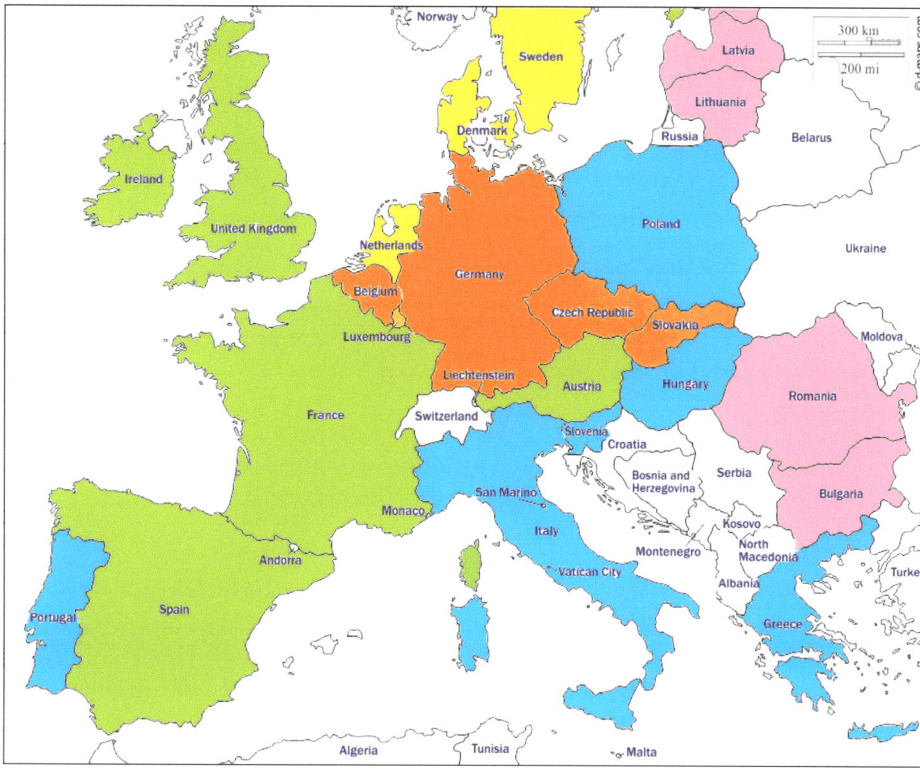

Figure 5.
Classification of LTC provision in EU. Legend: Yellow—Cluster A; Orange—Cluster B; Green—Cluster C; Blue—Cluster D; Pink—Cluster E.

Eligibility is defined by the high-care needs felt among the oldest cohort. This group of people not only has severe functional limitations but also has run-down most of their savings and assets. The package of services included in LTC needs to balance the cost and effectiveness of different modes of providing services. This may not be easy to assess. Some questions may then be raised, e.g., "how to decide what support is given to IADL?" or "how to decide to support in cash or in services?" Cost sharing is supposed to be based on the ability to pay; however, it may not be easy to define the fair share between public and individual responsibilities of pay. On the other hand, using saving and assets may be unfair as those individuals did not spend their money in past while others did.

The EU Commission [25] has suggested a typology of LTC provision for the EU members, enabling some international comparisons. This typology is built based on three criteria concerning the features of formal care. The first criterion is the organization of LTC which can be public, private, or non-for-profit. The second criterion corresponds to funding classified in general taxation, compulsory social insurance, voluntary private insurance, or out-of-pocket. Finally, the third criterion is provision which may take place at home or in an institution. Applying these criteria, it is possible to group the EU countries into five clusters, also presented in **Figure 5**.

- Cluster A (in yellow) includes countries with public provision of LTC financed by general taxes, low informal care, high informal care support, and modest cash-for-care benefits (Denmark, Netherlands, and Sweden).

- Cluster B (in orange) includes countries with medium public (mainly financed by compulsory social insurance) and low private formal care, high informal care and high informal care support, and modest cash-for-care benefits (Belgium, Czech Republic, Germany, Slovakia, and Luxembourg).

- Cluster C (in green) accounts for countries with medium public and private formal care (financed social insurance and general revenue), high informal care use and high informal care support, and high cash-for-care benefits (Austria, England, Finland, France, Spain, and Ireland).

- Cluster D (in blue) includes countries with modest social insurance against LTC risks; low public and high private LTC funding, high use of informal care but low informal care support, and low cash-for-care benefits (Hungary, Italy, Greece, Poland, Portugal, and Slovenia).

- Cluster E (in pink) group includes countries with little social insurance against LTC risks; very low public spending, very high informal care use but no support of it, and no or very low cash-for-care benefits (Bulgaria, Cyprus, Estonia, Lithuania, Latvia, Malta, and Romania).

Despite the funding criterion, clusters of countries include different mechanisms of funding LTC, both tax and social contribution based. So, clustering of LTC provision across countries in Europe may contribute to meaningful international comparisons of LTC policies, as well as the efficiency and fairness of funding strategies.

6. Sustainability challenges

Aging is expected to double public spending in LTC in the period 2010–2060. The current scenario of aging population and increasing of the LTC costs raises several challenges, including the question, "how to finance equitable and high quality LTC in fair manner?"

To assess this question, two overall challenges appear related to the sustainability of LTC under the UHC umbrella: first the financial sustainability and second the political and social sustainability.

The financial sustainability implies that there is some resource collection mechanism allowing a balance between the decreasing number of active people and the increasing number of elderly. Some countries have an underdeveloped LTC provision which makes financial sustainability a major concern given the increasing demand for LTC.

On the other hand, funding needs to be economic sustainable so that the share of GDP resources is collected and applied on LTC do not risk the country in a debt crisis. The funding mechanisms of health systems adapting to an aging society need to be carefully thought, in particular in countries where public debt is already a problem [18].

Second, political and social sustainability means that people in a country have decided and support how much they are willing to pay to finance LTC within UHC, in particular, to finance healthcare to those who are in need and cannot afford to pay for it [26]. Since complete universalism of LTC may not be feasible and trade-offs must be done, target universalism may be the most fair and efficient path to be chosen. The fairness of funding has to be not only intra-generational but also inter-generational. For target universalism to be successful, it has to be socially accepted and supported. This implies that the relative importance of social values is not dominated by economic values.

Informal care is a cornerstone of sustainable LTC provision, and it contributes to the financial sustainability. But informal care itself faces challenges related to care and attendance allowances, as well as opportunity costs for predominantly female informal care workers. These women need to be carefully considered in the system in order to make informal care possible to families [27]. On the other hand, informal care contributes to the closing gap between the fast increasing demand of LTC and the slow increase of its supply. The political support and the social sustainability of informal care are steps toward the implementation of the (target) universal LTC.

7. Conclusion

The aim of this chapter was to present the concept of universal health coverage and of long-term care and to discuss how it may be financed under the current scenario of demographic aging and increasing demand for long-term care.

Universal health coverage is the main aim of health systems all over the world. The achieved universalism is measured along three dimensions—breath, depth, and height of a UHC cube. Long-term care is one of the services provided by UHC, which needs rules of eligibility, of services provided, and of cost- sharing.

In a fast aging society, the importance of LTC is increasing. This means that funding should register a corresponding increasing funds collection. The difficult of LTC funding emerges because there are less and less people active contributing to the collective funds and more and more older people in need of LTC. This implies, first, the use of alternative forms of funding, which should be based on a large pool of individuals, and, second, the use of strategic purchasing and provider payment mechanisms.

The variety of LTC systems across countries makes comparisons difficult, so a possible classification proposed by the EU Commission is described in the chapter. Funding criterion does not dominate the clustering of countries. There are equally important features (organization and provision), which contribute to the characteristics of the LTC system.

UHC and LTC are expected to be sustainable and fair, and target universalism is a possible answer. The implementation of the desired health system needs to respond to sustainability challenges, either financial or socio-political. The response to these challenges will guarantee people access to LTC when needed in an equitable way, without suffering hardship late in their life years. So, not only a more active and socially focused leadership is needed across countries but also better governance is expected so that social values are considered with comparable weight as economic values.

Health systems being very complex in terms of demographic, economic, legal and regulatory, epidemiological, socio-cultural and political, and technological aspects, an improvement in one of these areas necessarily has an impact on a global improvement of the universality of coverage. Therefore, it is expected that governments strengthen these components of the health system to make it possible to achieve its goals and provide a high-quality healthcare. In economic terms, not to defend the universality of access, more than an ideological act, would be a serious economic error.

Conflict of interest

The authors declare no conflict of interest.

Author details

Aida Isabel Tavares[1,3]* and Pedro Lopes Ferreira[2,3]

1 ISEG-UL, Lisbon School of Economics and Management, University of Lisbon, Portugal

2 FEUC, Faculty of Economics of the University of Coimbra, Portugal

3 CEISUC, Centre of Studies and Research in Health of the University of Coimbra, Portugal

*Address all correspondence to: aitavar@gmail.com

References

[1] WHO. Resolution WHA58.33. Sustainable health financing, universal coverage and social health insurance. In: Fifty-Eighth World Health Assembly; 16-25 May 2005; Geneva. Vol. 1. Geneva: WHO; 2005

[2] UN. Road Map Towards the Implementation of the United Nations Millennium Declaration: Report of the Secretary-General. New York: UN; 2001

[3] UN. About the Sustainable Development Goal. 2015. Available from: https://www.un.org/sustainabledevelopment/sustainable-development-goals/ [Assessed: July 1, 2019]

[4] EU. Adequate social protection for long-term care needs in an ageing society. In: Report Jointly Prepared by the Social Protection Committee and the European Commission. Luxembourg: EU. 2014

[5] WHO. Arguing for Universal Health Coverage. Geneva: Switzerland; 2013

[6] WHO. Health Financing for Universal Coverage. 2019. Available from: https://www.who.int/health_financing/topics/benefit-package/UHC-choices-facing-purchasers/en/

[7] UN. World Population Prospects 2019. United Nations: Department of Economic and Social Affairs, Population Division; 2019. Available from: https://population.un.org/wpp/

[8] Bloom D, Canning D, Fink G. Implications of Population Aging for Economic Growth. NBER Working Paper No. 16705. 2011

[9] Fries J. Ageing, natural death, and the compression of morbidity. The New England Journal of Medicine. 1980;**303**:130-135

[10] Gruenberg E. The failures of success. Mills Memorial Fund Q. 1977;**55**:3-24

[11] Kramer M. The rising pandemic of mental disorders and associated chronic diseases and disabilities. Acta Psychiatrica Scandinavica. 1980;**62**(Suppl. 285):282-297

[12] Manton K. Changing concepts of morbidity and mortality in the elderly population. The Milbank Memorial Fund Quarterly Health and Society. 1982;**60**:183-244

[13] Eurostat. Expenditure for Selected Health Care Functions by Health Care Financing Schemes [hlth_sha11_hchf]. 2019. Available from: http://appsso.eurostat.ec.europa.eu/nui/show.do?dataset=hlth_sha11_hchf&lang=en

[14] Colombo F, Llena-Nozal A, Mercier J, Tjadens F. Help Wanted? Providing and Paying for Long-Term Care. OECD Health Policy Studies. OECD Publishing; 2011

[15] Evans D, Elovainio R, Humphreys G, WHO. The World Health Report—Health Systems Financing: The Path to Universal Coverage. Geneva, Switzerland: WHO; 2010

[16] Kutzin J. A descriptive framework for country-level analysis of health care financing arrangements. Health Policy. 2001;**56**:171-204

[17] Rodrigues R. Long-Term Care—The problem of Sustainable Financing (Ljubljana, 18-19 November 2014). Peer Review on Financing of Long-Term Care; Slovenia. 2014. Available from: http://ec.europa.eu/social/BlobServlet?docId=13220&langId=en

[18] Wouterse B, Smid B. How to finance the rising costs of long-term care: Four

alternatives for Netherlands. Fiscal Studies. 2017;**38**(3):369-391

[19] OECD. Growing Unequal? Income Distribution and Poverty in OECD Countries. Paris: OECD Publishing; 2008

[20] Fuchs VR. Economics, values, and health care reform. American Economic Review. 1996;**86**(1):1-24. Available from: https://web.stanford.edu/~jay/health_class/Readings/Lecture01/fuchs_health_survey.pdf

[21] Rubinstein A, Barani M, Lopez A. Quality first for effective universal health coverage in low-income and middle-income countries. The Lancet Global Health. 2018;**6**(11):e1142-43.

[22] Powell J, Menendian S, Ake W. Targeted Universalism: Policy and Practice. Haas Institute for a Fair and Inclusive Society. Berkeley: University of California; 2019

[23] Geyer J, Haan P, Korfhage T. Indirect fiscal effects of long-term care insurance. Fiscal Studies. 2017;**38**(3):393-415

[24] Kazungu KS, Barasa EW, Obadha M, Chuma J. What characteristics of provider payment mechanisms influence health care providers' behaviour? A literature review. The International Journal of Health Planning and Management. 2018;**33**:e892-e905

[25] EU Commission. Long-Term Care in Ageing Societies—Challenges and Policy Option. Accompanying the Document Communication from the Commission to the European Parliament, the Council, the European Economic and Social Committee adn the Committee of the Regions. Towards Social Investment for Growth and Cohesion - Including Implementing the ESF 2014-2020. SWD 41 Final. Brussels: European Commission. 2013

[26] Cheng TM. Universal Health Coverage: An Overview and Lessons from Asia. Harvard Public Health Review 4—Global Health. 2015

[27] Mosca I, van der Wees PJ, Mot ES, Wammes JJ, Jeurissen PP. Sustainability of long-term care: Puzzling tasks ahead for policy-makers. International Journal of Health Policy and Management. 2017;**6**(4):195-205

Chapter 4

Healthcare Coverage and Affordability in Nigeria: An Alternative Model to Equitable Healthcare Delivery

Alex E. Asakitikpi

Abstract

Healthcare delivery in Nigeria has faced major challenges toward achieving universal health coverage. While significant progress was made in the first two decades after the country's independence in 1960, the economic downturn resulting from the plummeting of oil price of which Nigeria was dependent led to a series of twists and turns in the health sector. Health policies were subsequently influenced by external forces, and the adoption of the structural adjustment program signaled a shift from a predominantly welfare scheme to the introduction of user fee and the resultant proliferation of private healthcare provision. This paper discusses the crises that followed the turbulent health policies ever since by identifying some key factors that were glossed over by successive government regimes in formulating health policies in Nigeria. The paper concludes by suggesting a more inclusive model that will ensure equitability in the health sector and accessibility to healthcare services in the country.

Keywords: Nigeria, health policy, healthcare coverage, universal healthcare, health-seeking behavior, healthcare delivery

1. Introduction

Health policies in Nigeria have undergone tremendous evolution in the past 60 years but without the desirable quality of healthcare delivery system in place to advance the health status of Nigerians. While successive governments have made concerted efforts to promote health equity and ensure unrestrained access to health services, majority of the citizens are still grappling with various health challenges. These challenges are copiously reflected in the current World Health Organization (WHO) statistics where maternal mortality is among the highest in the world accounting for 19% of global maternal deaths [1]. The estimate of infant mortality rate in the country is 19 deaths per 1000 births with mortality among children under 5 at 128 per 1000 [2]. Furthermore, the average life expectancy of Nigerians is estimated by the World Health Organization to be 54.4 with women having a life expectancy of 55.4 and men of 53.7 [3]. These dismal health indicators have necessitated the call from researchers and other stakeholders for the Nigerian government to consider creative ways of responding to healthcare issues in the country.

In an attempt to understand healthcare problems in Nigeria, two major schools of thoughts are discernible. The first supports the neoliberal health policy that anchors its philosophy on market forces and the introduction of user fee for the provision of health services [4]. On the other hand, there are others such as the Nigerian government who promotes the continued expansion of public health centers by introducing health insurance, which is supposed to insure patients at all times, thereby expanding coverage and accessibility [5]. While these positions have their merits and, in one way or another, have been implemented in the past six decades with little success, there are some salient issues that have been glossed over which militate against the successes of health policies in Nigeria as they have evolved over the years. In this paper, we discuss the shortcomings of earlier policies and argue that the lack of a proper understanding and contextualization of citizens' health needs and their health-seeking behaviors is critical in designing appropriate health policies in the country toward the provision of quality health and access to services to the generality of the population. We identify the shortcomings that are associated with the theoretical framework of previous policies and discuss the implication of these on healthcare provision in Nigeria. Finally, we propose a model that is all-embracing toward providing universal healthcare services to Nigerians.

2. Contextualizing healthcare delivery in Nigeria

For a proper understanding of the current health situation in Nigeria, it is expedient to historicize the evolution of its healthcare system and within that framework examine some of the pitfalls that are associated with various policies. Prior to the coming of Europeans to Nigeria, the indigenous peoples that make up the country relied entirely on indigenous herbal and fauna knowledge to resolve various health conditions. The healthcare system was based on the quality knowledge of practitioners as well as defined ways of apprenticeship to qualify as a healthcare provider [6]. The medical student was expected to go through years of training both in herbal knowledge, therapeutic processes, and psychosocial relations. The underlying principle of traditional medical system was a sacred calling toward the preservation of lives and to serve as a cohesive element in the society. While traditional medical practitioners may charge "fees" (in the form of barter and general reciprocity), this did not form the bases for practice as there was no fixed and clear-cut "cost" for services rendered. Within this reciprocal framework, medical practitioners were regarded as custodians of life and were accorded the utmost respect in the society. With the coming of Europeans from the fifteenth century and the subsequent introduction of Western medicine, healthcare services became monetized so that health services were rendered for a standard fee. Although the colonial government did not overtly introduce Western medicine to rural folks, the importation of Western-trained medical doctors as well as Western medicine coupled with the influx of missionaries that used Western drugs as a means of evangelism, the seeds of drastic change in traditional medicine were sown. One key factor that led to the undermining of traditional medicine and its subsequent neglect was the missionaries' association of traditional medicine with witchcraft, Satanism, and evil. By 1960 when Nigeria gained her independence, Western medicine had been firmly established in urban centers, while missionary activities had also penetrated some rural communities. It was this skeletal framework that incipient indigenous governments built on after independence.

The underpinning philosophy of the First Republic was to ensure that Western-styled healthcare delivery became the primary source of health service in the country, and in order to achieve this, the government invested heavily in health by awarding scholarships to indigenous students to study medicine, nursing, and other allied professions abroad. At the same time, the government of the day was also building hospitals (orthopedic, specialist, and general hospitals) both in capital cities in the states and in key urban centers. Equipping hospitals with personnel and consumables became the priority of the government. On their return from overseas, the early trained medical doctors were placed in key positions in the health sector, while the public was encouraged by the government to patronize public hospitals and Western pharmaceuticals that were provided free or heavily subsidized by the government. This welfare orientation of Nigeria's First Republic, incidentally, could not be sustained for long due to the downturn in oil price and the increasing corruption in political circles. The consequences of this development were dire: consumables became scarce commodities in hospitals, epileptic payment of salaries of health workers became the order of the day, and a deteriorating condition of service precipitated the mass exodus of medical personnel out of the country. At the same time, most health posts in rural and semi-urban communities were abandoned, and the rural folks who had initially had access to Western medicine and government generosity were left to fend for themselves. On the other hand, the patronage of Western medicine at the expense of traditional medicine had led to the dearth of highly skilled and knowledgeable traditional medical practitioners as most of them died without passing on their knowledge to the younger generation. Even if they had wanted to do so, it was difficult for them because majority of the younger generation had been introduced to Western education and religion (Christianity especially), which influenced their perception of traditional medicine as inferior to Western medicine and evil in their religious conviction. The confusion that these developments generated precipitated the rise of private medical practice both in urban centers and rural communities. The need to meet Nigeria's health challenges and the gap that was created by the exodus of qualified Western-trained practitioners as well as the dearth of skilled traditional medical practitioners paved the way for the proliferation of quacks and fake drugs from the 1980s onward [7, 8].

The introduction of private health practitioners led to the informal introduction of user fee in healthcare delivery and a concomitant rise in the cost of healthcare services. However, because of the economic downturn in the country starting from the late 1970s and the structural adjustment program that was initiated in the mid-1980s leading to the mass retrenchment in both the public and private sectors, fewer people could access private healthcare services [9]. This situation led to the massive importation of sub-standard drugs into the country. Furthermore, the breakdown of state machinery and the poor coordination of activities in the health sector encouraged unqualified personnel to set up health centers, quasi hospitals, chemist shops, and drug hawkers [10]. This situation generated an outcry for the complete overhaul of the health sector which culminated in the promulgation of Decree 34 of 1999 that established the National Health Insurance Scheme (NHIS).

3. Health-seeking behavior in Nigeria

The evolution of health policies in Nigeria has inevitably influenced the health-seeking behaviors of Nigerians. Incidentally, scholars who have examined health policies and their challenges in the country tend to lump the health-seeking behavior of the people and analyze it as a monolithic pattern [11]. On the contrary, however, patterns of health-seeking behavior in Nigeria are complex and multidirectional. Although economic analysts have classified Nigeria into two broad categories, namely, the super rich (the elites) and the masses, in reality, there are three broad groups: the upper class represented by the extremely wealthy including politicians, the middle class consisting of the working class urbanites, and the lower class comprising urban squatters and the rural masses. Even at that, in practical terms, there are still some finer divisions in these categories. For example, among the upper class are those that are extremely wealthy and, as a rule, do not receive medical treatments in the country, and this category may be referred to as the upper-upper class category. They travel out of the country for their regular checkup and for their medication. Those that occupy the lower upper class patronize both international (foreign) medical service and, for minor ailments, exclusive local private health centers.

The working class citizens who constitute the middle class also have sub-categories. Those who occupy managerial positions in the organized private sector, directors and director general in the public sector, as well as owners of medium-scale companies usually patronize exclusive private health centers within the country, while those who occupy the middle sub-category within the middle class patronize private health services and specialized hospitals (such as orthopedic and teaching hospitals) in the country. Those who belong to the lower middle-class category primarily access private hospitals as well as general hospitals. The majority of the lower class access state general hospitals, chemist shops, drug hawkers, and traditional health practitioners that are ubiquitous in the society. Theoretically, while this categorization may be useful for analytical purposes, the reality in Nigeria is that there is a lot of crisscrossing in terms of health-seeking behaviors so that even those who occupy the upper class also combine their foreign medical services with local and spiritual means which the lower class also patronizes. This convergence in health-seeking behavior should not be analyzed as monolithic as the quality of care received by individual groups differ significantly and, thus, have bearing on their overall health status. While those who occupy the upper class use traditional health or spiritual health service merely as complimentary to the health services they receive outside the country, those who occupy the lower class sometimes use spiritual home, traditional medicine as their primary source of healthcare either due to the unavailability of other forms of healthcare services or the lack of funds to access these facilities. These patterns of health-seeking behavior are partly influenced by the health policies that have evolved in Nigeria. This recognition as well as the beliefs of the people is significant in developing a more holistic health policy that will provide universal healthcare coverage.

While neoliberal healthcare reforms have succeeded in providing healthcare services both for the upper and middle classes, they have neglected or technically excluded the lower class, which constitutes the majority in Nigeria. The reforms that were carried out in respect of revamping the ailing health sector (re-equipping government hospitals, ensuring constant power supply, provision of Western drugs and other consumables) have mainly benefitted the upper class and the upper middle class. The restructuring and commercialization of these health centers mean a higher cost of accessing them which the lower class cannot afford [12, 13]. The same is true of the NHIS, which has as its primary focus on those who work in the public and organized private sectors. Overall therefore, the neoliberal reforms in the health sector tend to privilege the upper and middle classes and disempower those in the lower class who make up over 75% of the approximately 190 million citizens.

4. The challenges of neoliberal health reforms

The philosophical underpinning of neoliberal health reforms in Nigeria as elsewhere is anchored on the logic of market forces. Although not entirely new to

Nigerians, neoliberal framework has significant constraints in its applications in the country. The African health system, with its humanistic face and barter system, still demanded some form of reciprocity from patients and their households. The missionary hospitals also had some form of market orientation in its healthcare delivery system, and through the years Nigerians are well acquainted with paying for health services [14]. Despite the welfare scheme during the First Republic, majority of the citizens were still prepared to pay for health services when the state could not sustain its welfare scheme. With the proliferation of private healthcare and the importation of sub-standard drugs, which questioned the quality of healthcare delivery in the country, most people became weary of Western medical care and resorted to other forms of healthcare services including spiritual healing. If assured of high-quality drugs as well as quality healthcare services, most Nigerians will still be prepared to pay for these services. Despite the dislocation of healthcare systems leading to eclectic health-seeking behavior in response to the proliferation of healthcare services, most Nigerians especially those in the middle and lower class still have difficulties accessing these services due to their prohibitive costs and questionable quality of drugs. The World Bank's [15] estimates of over 60% of Nigerians living below the poverty line indicate that a significant portion of the Nigerian public cannot access quality health service due to the concomitant high costs that are associated with neoliberal reforms. Within this theoretical framework, majority of the Nigerian public are faced with a dilemma: either the government subsidizes for quality healthcare services for the majority of citizens to enjoy quality healthcare or the majority of citizens must access other forms of services with questionable quality. The government's efforts at restructuring the health system by providing funds for the rehabilitation of dilapidated hospitals and ensuring uninterrupted supply of quality drugs mean that costs of health services will inevitably go up. As reported by researchers [16], there is an inverse relationship between the cost of health service and patronage with the poor responding sharply to changes in cost of service. With such neoliberal reforms, the suspicion of the public toward the government regarding health services as experienced from the late 1970s only exacerbate their suspicion of the government regarding healthcare delivery and government's conspiracy to strip them of their citizens' right to quality health. This suspicion means that increase in health cost is translated as a conspiracy between local politicians, policy makers, and global economic forces represented by the international pharmaceutical industry. This conspiracy theory reverberates in most sections of the Nigerian society.

Besides cost, access becomes an important issue in discussing healthcare delivery within the neoliberal framework. As noted in the previous section, the structural adjustment program, which led to the reduction in health personnel and the abandonment of health centers in rural areas and semi-urban centers, meant that with the introduction of user fee, the ratio of health personnel to the population as well as the ratio of health centers to the population dramatically increased. On the other hand, the restructuring and rehabilitation of health centers led to more Nigerians in the upper middle and upper class reverting to accessing health services within the country, thereby pushing away lower middle-class members who hitherto accessed health services in urban centers. This disparity in healthcare accessibility is an important consequence of the neoliberal reform which skewed significantly those who have access to quality Western medical health services and those who do not. What this means is that the reforms initiated by the Obasanjo administration starting from 1999 only favored a few who occupy the highest echelon of the society and disempowered the majority of citizens. This scenario has left the majority of the citizens to seek for alternative healthcare services both in the informal private sector and the patronage of quacks and drug hawkers. The conclusion to be drawn from this assessment is that neoliberal reforms in the health sector did not succeed in providing universal health coverage and accessibility but succeeded in upgrading the healthcare system with a tiny minority of the population as its main beneficiary. The realization of this shortcoming prompted the federal government to initiate the NHIS with its cardinal aim of universal health coverage as well as accessibility and equity among the population.

5. Challenges of the NHIS

The philosophy behind the NHIS and its design seems promising especially in terms of equity and accessibility [10, 17]. Although a relatively new concept in the health sector in the country, insurance itself is not a novel phenomenon to Nigerians. The concept of insurance as it applies to various aspects of the Nigerian life has been in existence since the country's independence. But 10 years after the launching of the NHIS, no significant progress has yet been made. Only about 10% of the Nigerian population is covered by the scheme with the vast majority still left to fend for their health needs [18]. While the government has patted itself on the back for the modest progress in health insurance coverage, the reality is that most of the insured are private employees and government officials who are coerced to patronize the scheme. The exclusion of certain drugs and diseases such as diabetes, sickle cell anemia, HIV, cancer, and other chronic diseases also means that even those that are insured will seek alternative means to meet some of their health challenges. More importantly is the unwillingness of low- and medium-scale entrepreneurs to register their employees with the insurance scheme as stipulated by the Act. Entrepreneurs connive with their employees not to register with the NHIS as it is profitable for both parties to do so. The rationale behind this noncompliance is based primarily on the seeming benefits that both employers and employees believe they will enjoy since the Act mandates employers to pay 7.5% of the premium and the employees to pay another 7.5% of the total premium. The general belief is that registering for the NHIS would not guarantee access to quality health service due to various historical antecedents that are associated with insurance schemes in Nigeria [10, 19].

Various insurance schemes such as house insurance, education insurance, and life assurance that were introduced in Nigeria in the 1960s and early 1970s did not meet the expectations of those who embraced the schemes as their claims were not paid when the need arose. This disappointing experience led to the unofficial appellation of "pen robbers" that was associated with insurance companies. A similar case is the Nigerian pension scheme which also suffered a major scandal as a result of the nonpayment of retirees due to corrupt practices of government officials that were responsible in managing the pension funds. These historical experiences have significant bearing on the average Nigerian's perception regarding the sincerity of the government and the efficacy of its policies especially those that encourage contributions from the general public for a common good such as the NHIS. The government's alignment with global practice of neoliberal ideology is therefore seen by the middle and lower classes as a grand conspiracy by the ruling class to perpetuate the enormous gap between the elitist class and the masses. This conspiracy theory is grounded not only in the experiences of citizens in the health sector but in almost all facets of life in the Nigerian society. The gross neglect of the Nigerian public by successive regimes, starting from the mid-1980s, significantly eroded any confidence the people have in the government. It is precisely because of this disconnect between the state and its citizens that there is a lack of any meaningful social movement that forces the government to take up its responsibility and be accountable to the people [10]. In cases where professionals such as medical doctors, nurses, and other health workers have engaged in social protests such as strikes, the government of the day had handled such social protests with a heavy hand leading to the mass exodus of highly qualified personnel in the health industry, which further compounded the problem. The near collapse of the health sector in Nigeria is one of the most important factors for the proliferation of various cadres of healthcare services and the concomitant eclectic health-seeking behavior of Nigerians.

6. Healthcare providers in Nigeria

Various scholars who have discussed healthcare provision in Nigeria although have identified key healthcare providers in the country have failed to match these various providers with those that patronize them and why. Some scholars [20, 21] correctly dissected the various providers of health services in Nigeria which can broadly be classified into two groups: government-owned health centers and those owned by private organizations and individuals. While health services were predominantly provided by the government up to the mid-1980s, private health providers have exponentially increased in the last 30 years. Government health services are generally regarded as public hospitals and those owned by other groups as private, but this nomenclature may not be entirely correct in the twenty-first century and therefore may be misleading. It is true that before the introduction of user fees in government health centers, the general public had access to these health centers. However, the transformations of various government regimes initiated in the health sector have technically excluded majority of the public making it a "public-private" health center. On the other hand, private health centers such as hospitals and maternity homes that are owned by Christian missionaries although regarded as private have become more public than government-owned hospitals primarily because of the cost differentials between government-owned and missionary-owned hospitals. Furthermore, some of these missionary hospitals and maternities are sited in rural areas and semi-urban centers giving access to rural dwellers, thereby making the missionary hospitals more accessible to underserved communities.

In addition to the abovementioned forms of health providers is the proliferation of other healthcare providers, namely, the private hospitals that are owned by qualified medical practitioners, licensed pharmacists, the unqualified and unlicensed chemist shop owners, the ubiquitous drug peddlers, traditional drug hawkers, knowledgeable traditional herbal healers, and other forms of health providers including spiritual homes and churches. The high cost of accessing government specialist hospitals as well as teaching hospitals and the bureaucratic structure of general hospitals has increased the demand for private health provision, which predominantly caters for the middle-class cadre. Because of the availability of genuine drugs and the services rendered by private practitioners, the costs are generally high and are, thus, not easily accessible to the masses. Although the licensed pharmacist on the other hand sells genuine drugs, there are instances where some have engaged in sharp practices by mixing genuine and fake drugs or sometimes leasing out their certificates to unqualified personnel to set up chemist shops [7].

Incidentally, drug peddlers fill a unique gap in the health market as they source their drugs mainly from China, Thailand, India, and other Asian countries targeting a section of the population that is made up of unskilled and manual workers. The drugs that are usually sold include energy-boosting drugs, multivitamins, blood tonic, general pain killers, and other drugs that are associated with common health complaints associated with this group of people. The majority of customers who patronize drug peddlers are those in the low-income bracket, and although may patronize chemist shops, their major source of drug supply is through peddlers who also act as health advisers. These health "advisers" are usually strategically positioned in busy bus stops, marketplaces, and commercial busses. Traditional drug hawkers, like drug peddlers, also meet the need of specific categories of clients although sometimes the clientele spectrum cuts across economic classes. The traditional hawkers represent people who have some knowledge of traditional medicine or those who are recruited by traditional medical experts. Usually most of these traditional medicines are packaged in various forms (in bottles, wrapped in paper, nylon sachet, etc.) which are sold to the public. The illness types they target include children-related diseases (such as infections, diarrhea, skin rash, etc.), pile, eczema, dysmenorrhea, ring worm, poor sexual performance, and low sperm count, among others. This category of health providers enjoys large patronage primarily because of the low cost of the drugs and the cultural engagement the providers have with their customers. The cost of these traditional drugs is relatively cheap because they are locally sourced, while hawkers display a high level of familiarity with the drugs they sell and the diseases they are supposed to cure [22]. It is common to see these hawkers in strategic points such as crowded bus stops, marketplaces, and commercial busses (a major means of transport for low-income earners). They advertise their products with bull horns and other forms of public address systems to attract their audience. Sometimes they use patients who are suffering from ailments they claim their drugs can cure to demonstrate the efficacy of their products.

The marketing strategy of these hawkers is also displayed in commercial busses by engaging commuters first by praying in the local language and wishing everyone "Alafia" or good health. The hawker then proceeds by listing series of symptoms associated with a variety of diseases and then presenting their audience with the drugs that are applicable to cure the ailment. It is not uncommon to hear them discuss about Western medicines and their efficacy, but they are quick to also point out the high cost of purchasing them as well as the side effects they leave in the human body. This display of medical knowledge seems to be an effective way of convincing commuters to patronize their products. It is interesting to note that not only the uneducated public patronizes these traditional hawkers but the educated public also and some who belong to the middle-income class.

Often this category and the former category, namely, the hawkers of Asian drugs complement each other as it is not uncommon to see traditional medicine hawkers also selling Asian drugs. These two categories of health providers are the most common sources of healthcare service among the vast majority of low-income earners in urban centers, thereby occupying a strategic position in healthcare delivery in Nigeria. Skilled practitioners of traditional medicine although could be found in urban centers are predominantly the major source of healthcare in rural areas. They still retain the informal traditional structure of healthcare, but they have also introduced monetary rewards for the health services they render. While scholars have argued that traditional medical practitioners lack precise knowledge of diseases and have been criticized for the unhygienic environment in which they operate as well as lack of standardization of their therapy, they still constitute an important source of healthcare delivery in Nigeria. Although it is true that some practitioners do not have precise knowledge and skills to handle some form of ailments, credit must be given to them for their ability to treat common diseases and sometimes complex ailments such as mental illness, thereby creating stability in rural communities. Despite the general onslaught of medical practitioners and health scholars on traditional medicine and its practitioners, the fact remains that very few studies have been carried out to identify areas of relative strengths of traditional health practitioners. The general tendency of discussing traditional medicine as monolithic and unspecialized is grossly misleading and gives the erroneous impression that traditional medical practitioners are static in their knowledge and do not in any way improve upon the existing knowledge they received during their training. The policies have neglected these critical areas of healthcare provision, and the need to evolve some innovative ways of incorporating them into the overall healthcare policy must be initiated, developed, and executed.

Similar to the above, very few scholars have discussed the emergence and prevalence of religious and spiritual health centers and the role they play in healthcare delivery. These centers are different from missionary hospitals that were discussed above. By religious/spiritual health centers, we mean the rise of new religious movements (such as Pentecostalism and syncretic forms) as major providers of healthcare services that rely on patients' faith and spiritual leaders' ability to manipulate spiritual elements to achieve miraculous healing. By employing religious artifacts and relying on the efficacy of prayer for healing purposes, prophets and pastors encourage their congregation to combine faith with Western medicine or to wholly depend on the supernatural for their healing and miracles. Religious/spiritual health centers began to emerge as a major alternative source of healing in the 1980s. This is not surprising as it coincides with the period when the government public hospitals began to lose their appeal as a result of their neglect by the government. The patronage of this form of healthcare cuts across all spectrum of socioeconomic status. Those who patronize this form of healthcare, however, compliment the services with other forms of health provision; religious extremists completely rely on this form of healthcare for various ailments including child delivery and reproductive health more generally. These health providers may constitute a tiny minority, their influence is increasing, nevertheless, and they are attracting people from all cadre of the social strata.

7. Toward an alternative model for equitable healthcare delivery

The complex relationship between health-seeking behavior, the production and distribution of medicines, and health conditions in Nigeria requires a perceptive understanding of their interconnectedness and the development of an appropriate framework that will synthesize these patterns toward developing health policies that will reduce mortality and morbidity rates as well as improve the quality of life of citizens. The Nigerian government has not made significant progress in reducing maternal and child mortality as well as meeting the United Nations' health-related millennium development goals and the current sustainable development goals precisely because of this lack of coordination in the health sector. The neoliberal transformation in the health sector with its global perspective that anchors its principles on free market enterprise does not square with the sociocultural reality in Nigeria. While neoliberal reform took for granted basic social and economic factors in developing its structure and modalities, the neglect of these factors has far-reaching consequences in dealing with health issues in Nigeria. One of such sociocultural factors is the health-seeking behavior of citizens. In Europe and North America, response to ill health is essentially unidirectional and embraces Western medicine, but the same is not true in Nigeria as has been espoused in this paper. This is not to say that citizens in the West do not explore other forms of healthcare; what is essential is that they mostly utilize other sources such as yoga and acupuncture, among others, as complimentary medicines.

The conspicuous neglect in Nigeria's health policies in the variety of ways of seeking healthcare has greatly undermined the reality; hence the key principles of equity and coverage are severely compromised. Furthermore, the organic structure of the Ministry of Health even though has clearly defined hierarchy with local governments in charge of healthcare provision at the grassroots, state governments in charge of general hospitals in urban and semi-urban centers, and the federal government coordinating these tiers including tertiary health institutions and specialist hospitals, there is no officially recognized structure that coordinates other forms of healthcare providers. This lack of cooperation either at the federal or state government and the scattered informal healthcare providers is critical in understanding why various types of health providers with questionable skills and competence flourish in the country. This factor could be identified as the singular most important reason why mortality rates in Nigeria are still high especially in urban and semi-urban centers. On the other hand, mortality rates are also high in rural areas not necessarily because of the absence of state presence in these areas but because traditional medical knowledge has, since independence, been grossly neglected, thereby giving room for quacks to hijack by masquerading themselves as skilled medical practitioners. These traditional quacks and charlatans are primarily responsible for the high mortality rates that are recorded in rural communities. To overcome this challenge, the government needs to erect structures to coordinate the activities of skilled traditional medical practitioners and set up a formal standard to exclude quacks. In the long term, the government needs to set up research institutes that will encourage and support skilled traditional medical practitioners to document, research into the working models of traditional medicines, and explore ways of improving such knowledge. Since rural dwellers are comfortable with traditional medicine and because traditional healthcare practitioners have devised informal but effective ways of relating with patients in rural communities, government and medical research scientists need to explore these ways of patient-doctor relationship to serve as important innovations for policy implementation. Studies have shown that the formal and sometimes arrogant doctor-patient relationship in government hospitals is a significant factor why utilization is low [23–25]. Exploring this important dimension of healthcare provision and identifying alternative ways that are more culturally sensitive to the people will go a long way in achieving universal health coverage.

The recognition of African medicines and their practitioners by the WHO and its recommendation to African governments to adopt it in their health policy are in order, and there seems to be some progress made in this direction. For example, the number of African countries with national African medicine policies increased from 8 in 1999–2000 to 39 in 2010, and those with national African medicine strategic plans rose from 0 to 18. Countries' regulatory frameworks increased from 1 in 1999–2000 to 28 in 2010. Also, by 2010 eight countries had institutionalized training programs for African medicine practitioners [26].

However, despite the abovementioned progress, the issue of sustainability is still a recurring decimal in the analysis of healthcare provision in Africa. In Nigeria, as in other African countries, approach to healthcare sustainability still persistently tilts toward a global capitalist perspective which attempts to address this issue by encouraging the government to expand its budgetary allocation to the health sector for the supply of very expensive Western medicines that are beyond the reach of the average Nigerian. For example, the WHO has subscribed a minimum of 25, 18, and 14% at various times as the minimum budgetary allocation for healthcare. However, with poor economic craftsmanship, structural adjustment programs that were implemented in most African countries, corruption among government officials, and the competing needs of other sectors of the society have all undermined the ability of the government to sustain the huge cost that is associated with healthcare delivery. User fee experience in Africa toward the purchase of Western drugs indicates varied results. For example, Gilson [14] in her review of user fee experience on the continent noted that a significant number of African countries have not benefited from this kind of healthcare reform. Similarly, the review made by Lagarde and Palmer [27] regarding user fee experience in Africa indicates varied experiences with Nigeria having recorded mixed utilization rates. One reason for these mixed results is the complete reliance of African government on the importation of Western drugs and other consumables without a concomitant framework for the production of traditional medicines. The relative economic weakness of most African countries and their low GDP make it extremely difficult for African countries to sustain this expensive enterprise. As noted above, while Nigerians, especially those in urban centers, have embraced Western medicine and some can even afford it, majority of the citizens in rural areas as well as the urban poor are still comfortable with traditional medicine, and it is within their reach. There is a need therefore for the government to include in its health policy and within the ambit of the Federal Ministry of Health to encourage the local production and fair distribution of African medicines. Such herbal production should be closely monitored to meet the basic standards that the government will set for the purpose of quality control. Such efforts will not only create jobs for indigenous citizens, but more importantly, indigenous medical knowledge will also become fully developed and contribute to global herbal knowledge. Such projects when embarked upon will trigger a series of development within the country, one of such being the need to intensify campaign for faunal and floral renewal as these are the primary sources of traditional medicine.

The pervasiveness of religion in Nigeria and the increasing use of spirituality to meet health needs are critical in the healthcare equation even if not for curative purposes, but for therapeutic processes. Studies have shown that religion and spirituality are important coping strategies that patients use as part of their therapy. Studies conducted by Koenig [28] and in an extensive review of the literature [29] revealed a positive relationship between religion/spirituality and health outcomes; these results have far-reaching implications for healthcare delivery and health policy formulation in Nigeria especially so when almost all citizens have some religious affiliation and are spiritual in nature. Although still informal in the country, there are indications that both patients and providers actively seek the spiritual assistance of religious members as part of the therapeutic package. While this is a positive development, there is a need for the government to officially recognize this form of healthcare and incorporate it in its health policy for proper coordination.

8. Conclusion

Healthcare delivery has undergone tremendous transformation since Nigeria's independence in 1960. While significant progress was made in the first two decades, the economic downturn resulting from the plummeting of oil price of which Nigeria was dependent led to a series of twists and turns in the health sector. The structural adjustment program signaled a significant shift from a predominantly welfare scheme to the introduction of user fees and the subsequent proliferation of private healthcare provision. The chaos that followed this highly unregulated private healthcare and the introduction of fake drugs into the market precipitated an unprecedented maternal and child mortality as well as a general reduction of life expectancy in Nigeria. This chaotic situation led to the launching of the National Insurance Scheme that encouraged co-payment for healthcare services.

Although these efforts have recorded some gains, the result is still far from the expected target of the federal government which was to meet the MDGs. We have argued in this paper that the neoliberal reforms in the health sector, which is today epitomized in the NHIS, are defective in significant ways leading to problems of inequity, accessibility, and sustainability. While the core of the health policy may be maintained to continue to cater for the elite group in Nigeria, there is a need to expand the boundaries of the policy to accommodate and recognize other forms of healthcare service including indigenous healing practices and religious/spiritual healing by taking into consideration the complex nature of Nigeria's health-seeking behavior. Such expansion will not only reduce maternal and child mortality due to increase in accessibility and utilization, but more importantly, it will help to address the issue of sustainability. Generating drugs locally will meet the basic health needs of citizens especially those in rural communities, empower rural folks, and involve them as important stakeholders in the process of transforming Nigeria into a healthier nation.

Conflict of interest

The author declares no conflict of interest for this article.

Author details

Alex E. Asakitikpi
Monash University South Africa, Johannesburg, South Africa

*Address all correspondence to: alex.asakitikpi@monash.edu

References

[1] WHO. Trends in Maternal Mortality: 1990 to 2015. Estimates by WHO, UNICEF, UNFPA, World Bank Group and the United Nations Population Division. Geneva, 2015. Accessed from: https://data.unicef.org/wp-content/uploads/2015/12/MMR_executive_summary_final_mid-res_243.pdf Accessed [March 16, 2019]

[2] UNICEF. 2019. Available from: https://www.unicef.org/nigeria/situation-women-and-children-nigeria [Accessed: March 15, 2019]

[3] WHO. 2019. Available from: https://www.who.int/countries/nga/en/ [Accessed: March 15, 2019]

[4] WHO. Sustainable health financing structures and universal coverage. Report of the sixty-fourth World Health Assembly. Geneva; 2018

[5] Federal Ministry of Health. National Health Financing Policy. Abuja, Nigeria; 2006

[6] Ityavyar DA. Background to the development of health services in Nigeria. Social Science and Medicine. 1987;**24**(6):487-499

[7] Alubo SO. Death for sale: A study of drug poisoning and deaths in Nigeria. Social Science and Medicine. 1994; **38**(1):97-103

[8] Akinyandenu O. Counterfeit drugs in Nigeria: A threat to public health. African Journal of Pharmacy and Pharmacology. 2013;7(36):2571-2257

[9] Olukoshi A. Introduction: From crisis to adjustment in Nigeria. In: Olukoshi A, editor. The Politics of Structural Adjustment in Nigeria. Vol. 1993. Ibadan: Heinemann; 1993. pp. 1-15

[10] Asakitikpi AE. Healthcare targets and the national health insurance scheme limitations in Nigeria. African Development. 2016;**XLI**(4):29-45

[11] Chukuneke FN, Ezeonu CT, Onyire BN, Ezeonu PO, Ifebunandu N, Umeora MC. Health seeking behaviour and access to health care facilities at the primary level in Nigeria: Our experience. Ebonyi Medical Journal. 2012;**11**(2):51-57

[12] Alabi CT. Nigeria: Poor Nigerians Still Lack Access to Basic Health Care—Physicians. Daily Trust, 8 April 2018. Available from: https://allafrica.com/stories/201804090025.html [Accessed: March 16, 2019]

[13] Riman HB, Akpan ES. Healthcare financing and health outcomes in Nigeria: A state level study using multivariate analysis. International Journal of Humanities and Social Science. 2012;**2**:296-309

[14] Gilson L. The lessons of user fee experience in Africa. Health Policy and Planning. 1997;**12**(4):273-285

[15] The World Bank. Nigeria: Bi-Annual Economic Update: Fragile Economy. 2017. Available from: http://documents.worldbank.org/curated/en/349511494584937819/pdf/114996-WP-P163291-PUBLIC-NEUNoFinalfromPublisher.pdf [Accessed: March 16, 2019]

[16] Wang'ombe J. Cost recovery strategies: The sub-Saharan Africa experience. Paper presented at the international conference of the World Bank in Washington DC; 10–11 March; 1997

[17] Eboh A, Akpan GO, Akintoye AE. Health care financing in Nigeria: An assessment of the National Health Insurance Scheme (NHIS). European Journal of Business and Management. 2016;**8**(27):24-34

[18] Onyeji E. NHIS: Regulators should be Blamed for Poor Coverage of Nigerians—Official. Premium Times, Sunday, March 3 2019. Retrieved from: https://www.premiumtimesng.com/news/more-news/260920-nhis-regulators-blamed-poor-coverage-nigerians-official.html [Accessed: March 16, 2019]

[19] Edeh JN, Udoikah JM. National Health Insurance Scheme and healthcare administration in Nigeria: An assessment. International Journal of Social Science Research. 2015;**6**(4): 2383-2394

[20] Alubo SO. Underdevelopment and the health care crisis in Nigeria. Medical Anthropology. 1985;**9**:319-335

[21] Alubo SO, Hunduh V. Medical dominance and resistance in Nigeria's health care system. International Journal of Health Services. 2017;**47**(4):778-794

[22] Makanjuola AB. A cost comparison of traditional and orthodox mental health care. The Nigerian. Postgraduate Medical Journal. 2003;**10**(3):155-161

[23] Abiola T, Udofia O, Abdullahi AT. Patient-doctor relationship: The practice orientation of doctors in Kano. Nigerian Journal of Clinical Practice. 2014;**17**(2): 241-247

[24] Onotai LO, Ibekwe U. The perception of patients of doctor-patient relationship in otorhinolaryngology clinics of the University of Port Harcourt Teaching Hospital (UPTH) Nigeria. Port Harcourt Medical Journal. 2012;**6**(1):65-73

[25] Onotai LO. Inpatients' perception of doctors' attitude towards the management of their ill health in a Nigerian University Teaching Hospital. IOSR Journal of Dental and Medical Sciences. 2017;**16**(1):102-109

[26] World Health Organization. Progress Report on Decade of Traditional Medicine in the African Region. AFR/RC61/PR2, 5 July 2011. Available from: https://afro.who.int/sites/default/files/sessions/working_documents/AFR-RC61-PR-2-Progress-report-on-decade-of-traditional-medicine-in-the-African-Region.pdf [Retrieved: March 20, 2019]

[27] Lagarde M, Palmer N. The impact of user fees on health service utilization in low- and middle-income countries: How strong is the evidence? Bulletin of the World Health Organization. 2008; **86**(11):817-908

[28] Koenig HG. Religion, Spirituality and Health: The Research and Clinical Implications. 2012. Available from: http://www.hindawi.com/journals/isrn/2012/278730/[IPMC [Retrieved: March 16, 2019]

[29] Koenig HG. Religion, spirituality, and health: A review and update. Advances in Mind-Body Medicine. 2015; **29**(3):19-26

Section 3

Providing Quality

Chapter 5

Caring for Older People - Improving Healthcare Quality to Ensure Well-Being and Dignity

Sandra Pennbrant and Margareta Karlsson

Abstract

The aim of caring is to promote health. The global trend is that people are living longer, but in many cases, there is no support system for the care of older people, leading to major challenges in ensuring their health and well-being. The proportion of older people is expected to increase globally, and skilled healthcare professionals will be required to care for them. There is a risk that older people as suffering and vulnerable human beings will be forgotten due to the increasingly effective and technical care worldwide. A caring culture and relationship should be prioritised and developed to promote participation, well-being and dignity for older people in order to fulfil their care needs and ensure quality healthcare. It is important that research focusing on universal health coverage identifies the benefits of increased investment in service quality. To contribute to the improvement of this output, we propose the application of Eriksson's caritative theory. The aim of this theoretical chapter is to provide examples of how the dignity and well-being of older people can be promoted, at no additional cost to the person, by means of Eriksson's caritative theory, which can strengthen healthcare for universal health coverage.

Keywords: caring, dignity, healthcare quality, older person, universal health coverage, well-being

1. Introduction

Human beings' becoming in health and suffering can be both promoted and inhibited. Human becoming is characterised by life in a movement and to live means being in a constant movement of change and feeling of existence [1]. Nursing is of importance for improving and maintaining older people health [2]. As suffering human beings older people need to meet healthcare professionals who see and take responsibility for their suffering [3].

Ethical care for older people concerns being aware of their vulnerability and respecting them as human beings. In caring it is important to promote participation and focus on the older people's resources [4]. One study compared nursing home residents with community-dwelling older adults and found that older people in nursing homes were more depressed and that their well-being was impaired [5].

Professional care involves caring for a human being where the relationship differs according to the specific context. There is a risk that empathy and compassion can be lacking if the circumstances under which patients are cared for are continuously deprived of the necessary resources for high quality and safe care.

Relationships are of importance when caring for human beings. However, an ethics of care with a relational ontology is preferable [6]. When meeting other people, it is important to respect the dignity of the individual, especially in meetings with people who depend on others on a daily basis to cope with everyday life [7]. Nurses have a responsibility to treat all people with dignity and respect [2]. When caring for older people it is important that healthcare professionals confirm the older people's dignity as a human being and promote an experience of well-being in her/his complex healthcare situation. One way of promoting the older people's dignity and well-being is to use Eriksson's theory of caritative caring [8]. The aim of this theoretical chapter is to highlight Eriksson's theory for promoting older people dignity and well-being in the perspective of service quality of universal health coverage.

2. Older people care from a global perspective

The number of older people aged over 60 years is steadily increasing all over the world, thus their care and care needs will become an increasingly important part of healthcare. Improving the health and functional capacity of older people, as well as their social participation and security, is challenging for society [9]. The need for healthcare is universal and in the nature of care lies respect for human rights, including cultural rights, dignity, well-being and to be treated with respect [10, 11]. Older people want quality care. Despite this, the care they receive is not always perceived as respectful and dignified. In healthcare today, violations of the dignity of older people are common [12, 13]. A British study revealed that older people with a high sense of well-being live longer than their peers who are less satisfied. The study highlights the feeling of having a reason for existence as an independent factor with a strong connection to health. Care should not be focused solely on curing diseases but also on giving people the prerequisites for a meaningful life [14]. Health is a fundamental prerequisite for people's ability to achieve their full potential. For that reason, we need to invest in health by devoting resources to quality-assured healthcare systems, which implies that we are reinvesting in the development of society as a whole [15]. Caring for older people means providing qualified care and many do not receive the care they need [16]. Older people feel safe and secure with the healthcare they receive but believe that they are a low priority group [17]. There are no clear strategies for developing the care of older people in terms of how dignified and continuous care can be ensured [11]. Every person should have access to quality healthcare without risking financial difficulties. The challenge for many countries lies in determining how to expand healthcare to meet existing needs with limited resources. A cost-effective part of the solution is having motivated health workers [18], whose demeanour enhances the patient's sense of self-dignity and well-being.

3. Dignity in caring for older people

Dignity is related to human beings' body, soul and spirit. Absolute dignity means that each human being has inner freedom and responsibility for both her/his own life and that of others [3, 19]. The absolute dignity of the human being, i.e. the inner dimension, is free from values. Relative dignity, i.e. the external dimension, is influenced by the culture and context in which the human being is present. The human being has an absolute dignity that contains the spiritual dimension. Absolute dignity cannot be violated or taken away from the human being due to its indestructible holiness. The human being's duty consists of being in communion in reciprocity, love and service [19].

Relative dignity contains an inner ethical dignity that belongs to the spiritual dimension and an aesthetic dignity that belongs to the bodily dimension. Relative dignity depends on the human being's cultural values and is unique for each individual as it is based on her/his culture and situation [19]. Individualised care can confirm the human being's dignity [20].

Preserving dignity when caring for older people means individualised care, good treatment, listening, showing respect [21] and being well treated [22]. Autonomy, respect and dignity are important for enabling older people to live a dignified life in nursing homes [23, 24]. Dignity and self-esteem are promoted through respectful treatment, listening, giving choices and respecting privacy [25]. Safeguarding dignity also means taking the older people's perspective into account, i.e. personality, identity and self-determination. Being a unique person of value is important for human health and well-being [26]. An investigation conducted in Sweden revealed deficiencies in care because older people have to adapt to the care instead of the other way around. Having to adapt to the healthcare offered can be perceived as unworthy by the older person. The experience of dignity is crucial for the feeling of well-being [27].

Personal commitment on the part of healthcare professionals is required to get to know and confirm older patients [28]. The healthcare professional can confirm the older people's dignity by being present, showing pity and respect. In elder care, the older people's well-being can be strengthened by healthcare professionals enhancing her/his sense of meaningfulness in life. This achieved by creating different forums for connectedness that can strengthen the older people's self-esteem. In this way, the healthcare professional is involved in the older people's life situation [29]. To provide good care it is necessary to ensure that healthcare professionals receive sufficient education and support in understanding the concept of dignity, as well as the necessary resources to translate dignity into their everyday work [30].

4. Well-being in caring for older people

The concept of well-being is central in healthcare science and related to health, quality of life and life satisfaction [31]. Well-being describes how a person feels at a certain time and be a measure of happiness or misfortune [32]. Well-being and health are interlinked, and health is defined as a: "state of complete physical, mental, and social well-being and not merely the absence of disease" [33]. This means that health is not only a goal, but also a resource in daily life, and that well-being may contribute to health or to the maintenance of health [33]. From a healthcare science perspective, the body can be understood as being in a movement between health and disease, a habitation of well-being and suffering in the pursuit of dignity [34]. Health is thus achieved through a combination of physical, mental, emotional and social well-being. In this way, health involves well-being and physical, mental and social dimensions. Well-being is important for the individual's self-assessment, degree of autonomy, control and ability to manage the everyday environment [31]. The feeling of well-being is a condition where human beings experience their own health, regardless of illness or disability, which is an important human experience [7].

Well-being is a feeling, thus cannot be observed by others, while health is defined as a wholeness with soundness, freshness and well-being [35]. The use of a computer and the Internet can contribute to enhancing an older people's well-being, as factors such as learning, social benefits, participation and positive feelings have been identified [36]. The quality of life and well-being of older people are not only affected by health, but also influenced by other factors such as social and family relationships, social roles and activities [37].

In elder care, the older people's well-being can be strengthened by the healthcare professionals facilitating the rebuilding of her/his sense of meaningfulness in life. This can be done by creating different forums for connectedness, which can strengthen the older people's self-esteem.

5. Katie Eriksson's theory of caritative caring

One of the pioneers of caring science in the Nordic countries is Katie Eriksson. Her theory of caritative caring is also internationally known [8].

Caring consists of meeting the other with respect, warmth, honesty and closeness in time and space [8]. The fundamental motive for caring is love and healthcare professionals deeply want to do well, even if it is not always visible in their actions. A caritative approach means that care is an ethical act that involves taking responsibility for others. Caring ethics is feeling responsible for the other and a willingness to serve. The ethics of caring is constantly present and cannot be divided into parts. Good technological care is related to how well the art of care is performed [38].

Caring is an act performed in love. To convey love to another person means being generous and involves the people's basic attitude to life [39]. The starting point in caring is that there is something natural in every human being. The ability to nurture is developed in a favourable environment. Caring involves tending, playing and learning and includes the whole human being with body, soul and spirit. To care is to share and heal and has a health promoting purpose. The basic substance is always the same, even if the caring takes different forms [40].

Tending in caring refers to a concrete action of love and means confirming the other as a human being. It is characterised by warmth, closeness and touch. Play is important in caring due to the fact that it is an expression of achieving health, wishes and an art form in caring. Learning means developing as a human being and can open new possibilities [41]. Caring ethics implies seeing the reality as it appears to the patient and recognising her/his right to be confirmed as a unique person with an absolute dignity [38]. Non-ethical situations can, for example, be a slipshod piece of work, being heavy-handed, not respecting the people's right to be involved or not listening or taking account of the patient's integrity [42]. Love can provide possibilities to feel compassion and be involved in a communion with the suffering human being, while for the suffering person, knowing that there is someone who is present and remains close creates trust and makes the suffering less unbearable [43]. To share in caring means being able to participate, for example, share in feelings, experiences or how to distribute concrete work activities [44]. It is therefore important that Eriksson's theory has a clear structure. The structure must ensure visibility and clarity for healthcare professionals. In this way, healthcare professionals can work together with the older person in a social interaction to create a whole.

6. Eriksson's theory of caritative caring for promoting dignity and well-being in elder care

Eriksson's theory can be used when caring for older people to promote and strengthen their dignity and well-being, thus facilitating the provision of high-quality care.

In a caring relationship, caring ethics requires that healthcare professionals have the will to do well and treat the human being with respect and an absolute dignity, in addition to being willing to sacrifice something of themselves [8]. Caring for older people can mean that healthcare professionals are there for them, see and confirm their suffering and listen to their narratives. This can create trust in the caring relationships, leading to bodily and spiritual well-being. Through tending, playing and learning older people health process can be supported and maintained for a sustainable old age.

A caring relationship means that the human being must be allowed to be a person and confirmed in the care [20]. Caring means relieving a people's suffering through mercy, faith, hope and love. It manifests itself by tending, playing and learning in the caring relationship with the patient [3]. Caritative care is based on ethical decisions made to alleviate human suffering and becomes visible through thought, posture and action [27]. The person who suffers is in the midst of her/his own suffering and therefore needs to meet healthcare professionals who can confirm her/his suffering in nursing [3]. To be able to understand a patient who is suffering, healthcare professionals need to be able to see, confirm and invite the patient to a healthcare communion where there is the possibility to alleviate the suffering [45]. Care should be perceived as meaningful by the patient and what is meaningful should be felt in body, mind and spirit [3]. Dignity includes healthcare professionals' will and ability to see and respect the other's needs and desires. In the caring communion there is warmth and care. Security is created through healthcare professionals' ability to be present. When healthcare professionals protect the patient's privacy, they promote respect, responsibility, self-determination and equality [46].

6.1 Example of care actions that can promote well-being and dignity progressing towards quality service within universal health coverage

The condition for providing caritative care is that the healthcare professional uses her/his professional knowledge when she/he is part of a communion with the older person [47].

The care activity *tending* involves the older person being able to experience security in the form of reliability, where proximity and distance are respected by the healthcare professionals in the care relationship [7]. Tending care may involve the healthcare professionals maintaining trust, hope and bodily relief by the love in their hands and the warmth in their voices [34]. To increase the older people's sense of security in an unfamiliar environment, healthcare professionals can invite the older people's relatives to become involved in her/his everyday life. An additional factor in tending is that the older people have their own personal belongings around them, which can give the feeling of a home environment [7].

Through the care activity *play*, the older people's satisfaction can be enhanced by the fulfilment of needs and desires. The fact that the healthcare professionals employ a playful approach means that they have the ability to reconcile imagination with reality. To find the older people's health resources, healthcare professionals can encourage and support her/him by means of caring play where the activity is adapted to the people's needs and resources [7]. Healthcare professionals can use different symbols and metaphors to access the older people's inner world. Through this approach, they can contribute to the creation of a new reality for the older person in her/his situation, which can contribute to hope and reconciliation of the older person with the outside world [48].

The care activity *learning* is based on meaningfulness, preserving the older people's everyday habits and strengthening the feeling of a normal environment. Healthcare professionals teach the older person to preserve her/his life story, habits and interests [45]. The purpose of the care activity is to maintain the older people's life experiences and skills. In this care activity new understanding can be created, where strengths, resources and health barriers can be clarified, thus allowing the older person to gain a deeper insight into the self and the/her/his situation [48]. The care should be person-centred in order to create a meaningful everyday life for older people. The care activities of playing and learning can create a bridge between the body's reality and the possibilities of health [34].

The care activities *tending*, *playing* and *learning* can provide a meaningful everyday life for older people and be strengthened when healthcare professionals are educated, supervised and encouraged to reflect on these care activities. Through tending, playing and learning in caring, older people dignity and well-being can be promoted. To share in caring means being able to participate in feelings, experiences or the distribution of concrete work activities [44].

7. Closing reflections

It is in everyday care that the dignity and well-being of older people can be promoted for a sustainable life. To create a good relationship in the care of the older person, it is important to become aware of her/his suffering. Older people deserve care that is focused on their unique needs for dignity and well-being, and not what is most suitable for the healthcare professionals involved in their care. Understanding the vulnerability of the older person can provide nourishment in the care relationship. Seeing and meeting the older people's face and gaze can confirm her/his dignity and promote health. The nurse's responsibility to develop the care means that knowledge is harnessed to benefit the older person. Critical reflection on the activities together with others can lead to the elimination of inefficient care methods and ways of working. Healthcare professionals have the opportunity to create a high-quality care environment for older people with the help of Eriksson's caritative theory, which is viable in the global healthcare system. Healthcare systems should be concerned not only with disease and illness, but with supporting methods that are sustainable and effective in the long term for improving the health, quality of life, well-being and dignity of older people. In order to strengthen older people' well-being and dignity, at no additional cost, healthcare professionals can use the caring relationship model (see **Figure 1**). This model is a collaborative

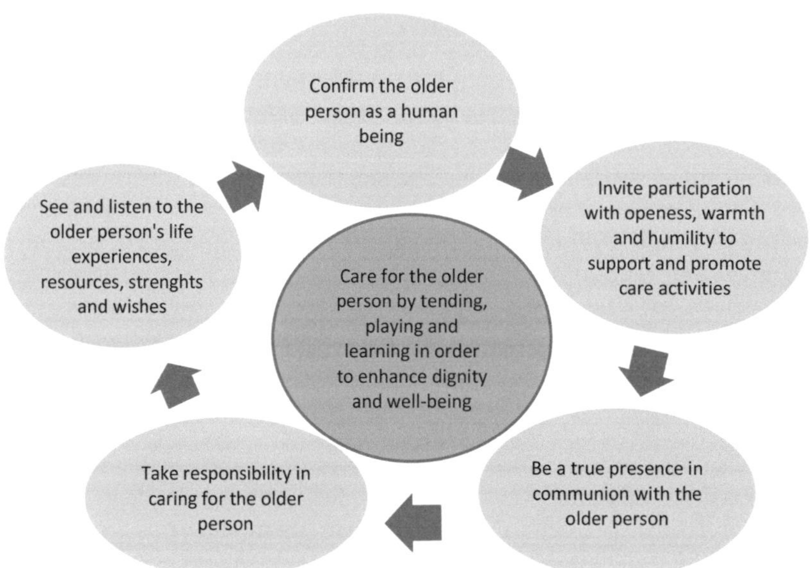

Figure 1.
An illustration of a model and process to improve the caring relationship activities of tending, playing and learning in order to enhance the quality of healthcare for older people, thus promoting their well-being and dignity.

process comprising five steps. The steps involve different approaches that healthcare professionals can employ to improve the care relationship activities of tending, playing and learning in the meeting with the older person by: (1) inviting the older person to participate in care activities, (2) communicating with true presence, (3) taking responsibility in the caring relationship, (4) seeing and listening to the older person's life story and (5) confirming the older person as unique with resources, needs and absolute dignity.

8. Conclusion

In order to improve the caring relationship with older people and to promote their well-being and dignity, it is important that healthcare professionals have the opportunity to use Eriksson's caritative theory combined with a collaborative process model. This theory and model are viable in the global healthcare system and can create national and international research networks to improve the coverage of health services within and between countries, and thereby promote a high-quality care environment for older people at no additional cost.

Conflict of interest

The authors declare that they have no competing interests.

Author details

Sandra Pennbrant* and Margareta Karlsson
University West, Trollhättan, Sweden

*Address all correspondence to: sandra.pennbrant@hv.se

References

[1] Nyström L. Hälsa, lidande och liv [Health, suffering and life]. In: Wärnå-Furu C, editor. Hälsans Praxis—I Liv Och Arbete [Health Practice—In Life and Work]. Stockholm: Liber; 2014. pp. 13-47

[2] International Council of Nurses (ICN). Ageing [Internet]. 2019. Available from: https://www.icn.ch/nursing-policy/icn-strategic-priorities/ageing [Accessed: Feb 12, 2019]

[3] Eriksson K. Vårdvetenskap Som Akademisk Disciplin [Caring Science as an Academic Discipline]. 3rd ed. Vaasa: Department of Caring Sciences, Åbo Academy; 2001. p. 80

[4] Høy B, Kloppenberg K. A dignity supporting elder care. Klinisk Sygepleie. 2012;**26**:4-14

[5] Cesetti G, Vescovelli F, Ruini C. The promotion of well-being in aging individuals living in nursing homes: A controlled pilot intervention with narratives. Clinical Gerontologist. 2017;**40**:380-391. DOI: 10.1080/07317115.2017.1292979

[6] Nortvedt P, Hem MH, Skirbekk H. The ethics of care: Role of obligations and moderate partiality in health care. Nursing Ethics. 2011;**18**:192-200

[7] Eriksson K. Hälsans Idé [The Idea of Health]. 2nd ed. Stockholm: Liber; 1993. p. 146

[8] Lindström UÅ, Lindholm L, Zetterlund JE. Katie Eriksson: Theory of caritative caring. In: Marriner-Tomey A, Alligood MR, editors. Nursing Theorists and Their Work. 7th ed. USA: Missouri, Mosby Elsevier; 2010. pp. 191-221

[9] World Health Organization. World Report on Ageing and Health [Internet]. 2015. Available from: https://www.who.int/ageing/events/world-report-2015-launch/en/ [Accessed: Feb 12, 2019]

[10] United Nations. World Population Ageing 2013 [Internet]. 2013. Available from: www.un.org/en/development/desa/population/publications/pdf/ageing/WorldPopulationAgeing2013.pdf [Accessed: Feb 12, 2019]

[11] Svensk Sjuksköterskeförening. Äldre Personers Rätt Till Omvårdnad—Behov, Kompetenser, Myter och Evidens [Older People's Right to Nursing Care—Needs, Competences, Myths and Evidence]. Stockholm: Sweden; 2014. p. 22

[12] SOU. Värdigt Liv i Äldreomsorgen [Dignified Life in Elder Care]. Vol. 51. Stockholm: Fritzes; 2008. 367 p

[13] Jakobson R, Sørlie V. Dignity of older people in a nursing home: Narratives of care providers. Nursing Ethics. 2010;**17**:289-300. DOI: 10.1177/0969733009355375

[14] Steptoe A, Deaton A, Stone AA. Subjective wellbeing, health, and ageing. Lancet. 2014;**14**:640-648. DOI: 10.1016/S0140-6736(13)61489-0

[15] United Nations. Transforming our world: The 2030 agenda for sustainable development. A/RES/70/1 [Internet]. 2015. Available from: https://sustainabledevelopment.un.org/index.php?page=view&type=400&nr=2125&menu=1515 [Accessed: Feb 3, 2019]

[16] Nordam A, Torjuul K, Sörlie V. Ethical challenges in the care of older people and risk of being burned out among male nurses. Journal of Clinical Nursing. 2005;**14**:1248-1256. DOI: 10.1111/j.1365-2702.2005.01230.x|

[17] Werntoft E, Hallberg RI, Edberg A. Older people's reasoning about age-related prioritization in health care. Nursing Ethics. 2007;**14**:399-412

[18] World Health Report 2013: Research for universal health coverage [Internet]. 2013. Available from: https://www.who.int/whr/en/ [Accessed: Feb 18, 2019]

[19] Edlund M. Människans värdighet—ett grundbegrepp i vårdvetenskapen [Human dignity: A basic caring science concept] [thesis]. Department of Caring Science, Åbo Academy University; 2002

[20] Eriksson K. Lidandet i vården [The Suffering in the Care]. In: Eriksson K, editor. Vårdvetenskap. Vetenskapen om Vårdandet och det Tidlösa i Tiden [Caring Science. The Science of Caring and the Timeless in Time]. Stockholm: Liber; 2018a. pp. 384-399

[21] Anderberg P, Berglund A, Lepp M, Segesten K. Preserving dignity in caring for older adults: A concept analysis. Journal of Advanced Nursing. 2007;**59**:635-643. DOI: 10.1111/j.1365-2648.2007.04375.x|

[22] Anderberg P. Bevarad värdighet i vård av äldre personer på äldreboende [preserved dignity in the care of older people in a nursing home] [thesis]. Karlstad: Karlstad University Studies; 2009

[23] Slettebö Å, Haugen Baunch E. Solving ethically difficult care situations in nursing homes. Nursing Ethics. 2004;**11**:543-552

[24] Teeri S, Leino-Kilpi H, Välimäki M. Long-term nursing care of elderly people: Identifying ethically problematic experiences among patients, relatives and nurses in Finland. Nursing Ethics. 2006;**13**:116-129

[25] Woolhead G, Calnan M, Dieppe P, Tadd W. Dignity in older age: What do older people in the United Kingdom think? Age and Ageing. 2004;**33**:165-170

[26] Eriksson K, Lindström U. Gryning—En Vårdvetenskaplig Antologi [Dawn—A Care Scientific Anthology]. 1st ed. Åbo: Åbo Akademins Förlag; 2000. p. 175

[27] Söderlund M. Som drabbad av en orkan. Anhörigas tillvaro när en närstående drabbas av demens [As if Struck by a Hurricane: The Situation of the Relatives of Someone Suffering from Dementia] [thesis]. Department of Caring Science, Åbo Academy University; 2004

[28] Franklin LL, Ternestedt BM, Nordenfelt L. Views on dignity of elderly nursing home residents. Nursing Ethics. 2006;**13**:130-146

[29] Näsman Y. Hjärtats vanor, tankens välvilja och handens gärning—dygd som vårdetiskt grundbegrepp [habits of the heart, benevolence of the mind, and deeds of the hand—virtue as a basic concept in caring ethics] [thesis]. Department of Caring Science, Åbo Academy University; 2010

[30] Gallagher A, Lee D, Li S, Rees Jones I, Wainwright P. Dignity in the care of older people—A review of the theoretical and empirical literature. BMC Nursing. 2008;7:11. DOI: 10.1186/1472-6955-7-11

[31] Dehlin O, Hagberg B. Gerontologi: Åldrandet i ett Biologiskt, Psykologiskt och Socialt Perspektiv [Gerontology: Aging in a Biological, Psychological and Social Perspective]. 1st ed. Sweden: Falköping: Natur och Kultur; 2000. p. 320

[32] Nordenfelt L. Livskvalitet och Hälsa—Teori och Praktik [Quality of Life and Health—Theory and Practice]. 2nd ed. Linköping: The Tema Institute, Health and Society. Linköping University, Faculty of Arts and Sciences; 2004. p. 160

[33] World Health Organisation. Constitution of the World Health Organization. New York: WHO, International Health Conference

[Internet]. 1946. Available from: https://www.who.int/governance/eb/who_constitution_en.pdf [Accessed: Feb 12, 2019]

[34] Lindwall L. Kroppen som bärare av hälsa och lidande [The Body as a Carrier of Health and Suffering] [thesis]. Department of Caring Science, Åbo Academy University; 2004

[35] Eriksson K. Hälsa är sundhet, friskhet och välbefinnande [Health is healthiness, freshness and well-being]. In: Eriksson K, editor. Vårdvetenskap. Vetenskapen om Vårdandet och det Tidlösa i Tiden [Caring Science. The Science of Caring and the Timeless in Time]. Stockholm: Liber; 2018b. pp. 152-165

[36] Shapira N, Barak A, Gal I. Promoting older adults' wellbeing through Internet training and use. Aging & Mental Health. 2007;**11**:477-484

[37] Dolan P, White MP. How can measures of subjective well-being be used to inform public policy? Perspective Psychology Sciences. 2007;**2**:71-84

[38] Eriksson K. Mot en caritativ vårdetik [Towards a caritative ethics]. In: Eriksson K, editor. Mot en Caritativ Vårdetik. Department of Caring Sciences, Åbo: Åbo Academy; 1995. pp. 9-39

[39] Eriksson K. Caritas tanken—människokärleken som vårdvetenskapens kunskapsobjekt [The idea of caritas—human love as the knowledge object of care sciences]. In: Eriksson K, editor. Vårdvetenskap. Vetenskapen om Vårdandet och det Tidlösa i Tiden [Caring Science. The Science of Caring and the Timeless in Time]. Stockholm: Liber; 2018. pp. 445-456

[40] Eriksson K. Vårdandets idé och ursprung [The idea and origin of caring]. In: Eriksson K, editor. Vårdvetenskap. Vetenskapen om Vårdandet och det Tidlösa i Tiden [Caring Science. The Science of Caring and the Timeless in Time]. Stockholm: Liber; 2018. pp. 237-239

[41] Eriksson K. Vårdsubstansen—att ansa, leka och lära [Care substance-to tend, play and learn]. In: Eriksson K, editor. Vårdvetenskap. Vetenskapen om Vårdandet och det Tidlösa i Tiden [Caring Science. The Science of Caring and the Timeless in Time]. Stockholm: Liber; 2018. pp. 245-257

[42] Herberts S, Eriksson K. Vårdarnas etiska profil [Caring ethical profile]. In: Eriksson K, editor. Mot en Caritativ Vårdetik [Nurses Ethical Profile. Towards a Caritative Caring Ethics]. Department of Caring Sciences, Åbo Academy; 1995. pp. 41-62

[43] Eriksson K. Den Lidande Människan [The Suffering Human Being]. 2nd ed. Stockholm: Liber; 1994. p. 112

[44] Eriksson K. Att vårda är att dela [To nurture is to share]. In: Eriksson K, editor. Vårdvetenskap. Vetenskapen om Vårdandet och det Tidlösa i Tiden [Caring Science. The Science of Caring and the Timeless in Time]. Stockholm: Liber; 2018f. pp. 263-266

[45] Söderlund M. Mänsklig värdighet i vården [Human dignity in health care]. In: Eriksson K, Lindström UÅ, editors. Gryning en Vårdvetenskaplig Antologi [Dawn a Care Scientific Anthology]. Department of Caring Sciences, Åbo: Åbo Academy; 2000. pp. 141-159

[46] Frilund M. En vårdvetenskaplig syntes mellan vårdandets ethos och vårdintensitet [A synthesizer of Caring science and nursing intensity] [thesis]. Vasa: Oy Arkmedia; 2013

[47] Eriksson K. Pro Caritate. En Lägesbestämning av Caritativ Vård

[A Situational Determination of Caritative Care]. 3rd ed. Vasa: Department of Caring Sciences, Åbo: Åbo Academy; 1990. p. 122

[48] Malm M. Själen [The soul]. In: Wiklund Gustin L, Bergbom I, editors. Vårdvetenskapliga Begrepp i Teori Och Praktik [Concepts of Caring Science in Theory and Practice]. 2nd ed. Stockholm: Liber; 2012. pp. 144-154

Chapter 6

An Intersectional Innovative Analysis of How Providers' Discourses Interact with Universal Healthcare Access

Lorena Saletti-Cuesta and Lila Aizenberg

Abstract

Intersectionality is an analytical tool for understanding the ways gender intersects with and is constituted by other social factors such as social class, age, and ethnicity, among others. The chapter discusses the theoretical and analytical intersectionality perspective, focusing on its application to an analysis of empirical data obtained from qualitative research. Semi-structured interviews took place with healthcare providers in Cordoba, Argentina. Thematic analysis was conducted. The findings show the existence of multiple domination systems incorporated in providers' discourses. All of them interact and contribute to gender inequalities in health, specifically on women's access to universal healthcare for violence against women and/or health of migrant women increasing their vulnerability. Training and sensitization among providers regarding gender and health from an intersectional approach are highly recommended as the first step toward a better healthcare system response.

Keywords: intersectionality, gender, access to health, qualitative methodology, healthcare providers, migration, migrant's healthcare, violence against women

1. Introduction

Intersectionality has increasingly been applied to health system research, especially works that aim to understand and respond to how multifaceted power structures and process produce and sustain health inequalities [1, 2]. Emerged from black feminist thought and first formulated by American sociologist Kimberlé Crenshaw in 1989 [3], intersectionality moves researchers beyond understanding individuals' unique circumstances and identities toward considering the drivers of inequality and to examining power relations at both individual and macro levels. Intersectionality challenges practices that privilege any specific form of inequality, such as race, ethnicity, class, or gender, and emphasizes the potential of different configurations of social locations and interacting social processes in the production of such inequities.

Intersectionality approach has been applied to healthcare studies and health inequalities to achieve two crucial aims. First, it brings attention to relevant differences within population groups that are often portrayed as relatively homogenous

 IntechOpen

such as migrants, indigenous people, or healthcare professionals. For example, it sheds light to an understanding that a white poor woman might be discriminated for her gender and class status when accessing healthcare but has the relative advantage of ethnicity or race over an indigenous or migrant woman. Second, it highlights the fact that health outcomes resulted from power structures of social domination and historical discriminations [4].

Thus, intersectionality moves beyond examining individual factors of health inequities such as biology, socioeconomic status, sex, age, gender, and race or the sum of them. On the contrary, it focuses on the relationships and interactions between such factors and across multiple levels of society to determine how gendered inequalities intersect with other aspects of oppressions that include not just gender but multiple social dominations [5]. Gendered inequalities thus intersect with other aspects of oppression, resulting in unique constellations that include not just gender but race, sexuality, ability, age, social class, caste, or position as a citizen, indigenous person, and refugee, among others. For example, an undocumented migrant will have qualitatively different experiences from a migrant who holds citizenship status.

Therefore, intersectionality has the potential to enrich public health research through improved validity and greater attention to both heterogeneity of effects and causal processes producing health inequalities [5]. As an overarching concept, intersectionality has much to offer to population health in providing a more precise identification of inequalities, in developing intervention strategies, and in ensuring that results are relevant within specific communities. Moreover, it was recently identified as an important theoretical framework for public health [6], as well as for gender and health studies [7].

To illustrate the relevance of intersectionality on understanding providers' discourses, we consider two important health issues on women's access to universal healthcare: violence against women and health of migrant women.

It is well-known that violence against women is an extreme manifestation of gender inequity, targeting women and girls because of their subordinate social status in society [8, 9]. In its multiple forms, it is recognized as a global healthcare problem and a serious violation of women's rights [10–13]. Moreover, violence affects women in different ways, particularly their health [14–16]. Therefore, healthcare systems have a crucial role in detecting, referring, and caring for women affected by violence [17]. A recent systematic review has explored primary care providers' opinions and experiences of tackling violence against women. The findings show that providers hold a range of opinions on the causes of violence against women. For example, some primary care providers perceived violence as a private matter mainly caused by relationship problems, drug abuse, or unemployment. Therefore, there is a need to better understand the social gendered roots of violence against women [18]. This is important considering that healthcare providers frequently, and often unknowingly, encounter violence among their users.

On the other hand, the increasing participation of women in migration processes, the growing tendency to incorporate gender approaches in the social sciences, and the conceptual opening to the figure of the migrant woman [19] have shown that migration processes are complex phenomenon shaped considerably by gender relations [20]. Social sciences have highlighted the need to approach the dynamic intersection between the different components present in the historical structures of domination [21, 22]. Social science analyses have demonstrated the value of the intersectionality of gender dimensions, ethnicity, social class, and national origin in migration studies [23] and the outcomes of the interactions of the categories which, in the case of female migrants, are placed in the social periphery. This has led to a growing attention to the relationships between migration;

intra-family dynamic, social contexts of women; impacts of displacement on gender roles; and migration outcomes on the quality of life of women, including their sexual and reproductive health [24].

Migration is, therefore, recognized as a key determinant of health [4]. For example, compared to their native counterparts, migrant women experience a higher number of unwanted pregnancies and report lower use of contraceptives and a lower propensity to attend reproductive health services in Latin America [25]. In this sense, migration has been identified as a risk factor, showing that the confluence of gender, ethnicity, and nationality and the lack of official citizenship documents can lead to the most extreme human rights violations, including sexual abuse, deterioration of reproductive health, and threats to physical integrity [26].

In the specific case of women, migrants are even more exposed to encountering obstacles to healthcare services. In addition to the difficulties they have as migrants, women face obstacles due to factors associated with their social class, gender, and ethnic-cultural background [27]. Despite these factors, studies have overemphasized cultural differences between migrant populations and the health system as relationships based on distrust among professionals and users due to cultural gaps [28]. This is why intersectional lens are crucial to understand multilevel factors shaping healthcare provision, practices, and use among migrant groups [4].

This article aims to include intersectionality theory to better understand the multiple axes of inequalities that cross healthcare providers' discourses on violence against women and health problems of migrant women. Intersectional lens becomes a promising approach to highlight the limits to health research and healthcare responses to migration and violence against women that overemphasize a single causal element of health outcomes—such as cultural differences or class—while highlighting multiple factors that shape healthcare views and healthcare practices in Argentinian healthcare system.

2. Method

This qualitative study was conducted in two phases in Cordoba, Argentina.

In phase one, healthcare providers from primary care centers or a regional hospital from urban and semi-urban regions of Cordoba were recruited using purposive sampling. Data were collected in different periods from June 2013 to November 2016.

In phase two, we used purposive sampling to recruit healthcare providers who worked in primary care centers or in a regional hospital from a semi-urban northern region of Cordoba. Professionals with least than a year of experience working in the setting were excluded. Data were collected over a period of 15 months from November 2016 to February 2018.

In both phases semi-structured interviews were conducted. All interviews were conducted by the authors. The interview guides used in each phase were pilot tested. It included basic sociodemographic information. In phase one the guide included questions that gathered their perceptions regarding migrant populations in general and the Bolivian flow in particular, as well as the existing barriers and facilitators in the access and use of health services by migrant women. In phase two the questions focused on four main topic areas: violence against women's opinions, experiences, barriers to provide care, and ways to overcome these obstacles. The interviews were conducted during regular working hours in a private place located in the health center or in the hospital. Each interview lasted ~60 minutes. They were audio recorded and transcribed verbatim for analysis. Full signed and informed consent was gained from all participants. Ethical approval was obtained through the College of Psychologists of Cordoba.

Inductive thematic analysis was conducted following Braun and Clarke's method [29] for identifying, analyzing, and reporting patterns (themes) within data. Transcripts of each phase have been reviewed independently by the researchers in an iterative process with the following stages: familiarization with the data, production of initial codes from the data, identifying themes, reviewing themes, and defining and naming themes. Saturation was achieved within the themes and categories. When all of the transcripts from each phase were coded and analyzed, the investigators met to reorganize them all into meaningful themes focusing on intersectionality and taking into account sociodemographic information. As Anuj Kapilashrami and Olena Hankivsky [4] mentioned, there is no single way to approach intersectionality and no preferred method. However, the authors recognized the importance of interpreting the commonalities and differences within and across population groups without being reductionists and linking individual levels of experience to social structures of power. This last stage resulted in an organized and comprehensive summary of multiple domination systems incorporated in providers' discourses. ATLAS.ti version 7.5.4 was used to help with management of the data.

A total of 50 providers (39 female and 11 male) participated in the research aged 30–59 years. They were from five communities (three from northern Cordoba, one from the center of Cordoba, and one from the periphery of Cordoba City). Regarding their professions, 20 of them were physicians, 13 nurses, 8 psychologists, 6 social workers, 2 dentists, and 1 radiologist.

3. Violence against women

The opinions of the healthcare providers regarding violence against women were varied and show how multiple factors shape healthcare opinions and practices contributing, some of them, to gender inequalities.

A mutual couple conflict, being in an unhealthy couple relationship, no respect, or lack of values were the root causes of violence against women according to the majority of healthcare providers. From this point of view, violence was as a private/domestic matter, making either men or women responsible for violence. For some providers interviewed, both members of the couple were considered "sick." From their point of view, these "unhealthy links" would cause a vicious circle between both members. Moreover, due to the naturalization of the violence, it was difficult to identify certain acts as violence and, therefore, to break circle of violence, according to providers' points of view.

> *"From my medical point of view, I believe that it is a disease of both. I think probably he has previously gone through other situations and came to this one...." (Woman physician, hospital)*

> *"The violence starts with the values, the limits, the culture that they receive, first from the family, the school, the social environment... We always see the last part of the film, when we have to act ... with someone already physically or psychologically injured. But we see the end, almost the end, because that story started many years ago. Why a person becomes an aggressor, becomes violent with another, and why that other one did not respond to stop that violence and accepts and justifies it...We works with two sick people...." (Men physician, primary care)*

This psychologization of the problem is a way of reducing a complex social problem to an individual or couple's disorder or conflict, which would reveal that the health sector does not correctly address the problem of violence against women by not understanding it as a multifaceted phenomenon that is produced by the complex interaction of individual, relational, community, and social factors [30, 31]. Also, they defined violence against women as a pathology or a defect. Understanding violence as a sign of disease reveals biomedical conception of health and places the health sector in an active and expert role. From this place, healthcare providers would have the knowledge/power on how the relationships between men and women "should be." Healthcare providers have been trained to investigate and diagnose a disease, to solve a problem, and to help their patients. However, in the case of violence against women, this role must be left aside to focus on the needs of patients, giving them a leading role in the decision-making process [32].

On the other hand, several people interviewed consider that women, mainly from vulnerable sectors, were partly responsible for their situation of violence since, from their perspective, they are also "sick" and justified the mistreatment they receive. These ideas not only release men from their responsibility but also contribute to normalizing violence against women by blaming vulnerable women for remaining in situations of violence [33]. It has been pointed out that not knowing about violence against women not only could hinder professionals to not inquire about this problem [18, 34] but also could influence women's trust in professionals [35], which contributes to perpetuate this serious problem.

This is important because it is related to how providers understand women as victims of violence and the barriers that prevent women from reporting their situation. For instance, some providers highlighted women's tendencies to hide abuse, low self-esteem, lack of family support, economic dependency, and social isolation, as well as their feelings of shame, guilt, or insecurity, their own acceptance of traditional gender roles, or their fear of social stigmatization.

Moreover, violence against women was understood as a patron of behavior transmitted from generation to generation. From providers' opinions, lacking values and limits, especially in childhood, childhood abuse, and/or violence experienced in childhood within the family context would explain why men perform violence in their adult life and also why women choose violent couples and justify their violence.

> *"...it is always repeating, things that have happened as a child they will do it again and so...afterwards it will happen later with the creatures raised in that family. It will continue, it seems to me. There is a lack of education, of emotional contention." (Woman radiologist, hospital)*

> *"Mainly that women become aware and take conscience of the situation... I think it will take a long-term work, I would tell you from the time they are girls, from elementary school, to do a raising awareness work focusing on women to show them that this situation is not normal, even though they see it at their homes: my dad hit my mom or spit on her, or insulted her, and those situations goes unnoticed. It is important that girls become aware that violence is not good... so they are clear about what is right and what is wrong." (Men physician, hospital)*

These opinions stated families not only as a power structure but also as the main agent of socialization that produce and sustain violence and gender disparities. This belief could be an important barrier to understand violence against women as a multifactorial phenomenon that is part of the patriarchal social structure where all social agents are responsible for its maintenance and reproduction, including the health sector [36].

Moreover, social class bias underlined providers' ideas about family models, violence, and education illustrating how various factors are affecting providers' opinions and practices simultaneously. Belonging to the working class was a risk factor for violence against women, according to some providers.

> *"It is very difficult for the victim of violence to get out of that situation and when she does sometimes, she not has a supportive family network... she not has the resources...it is very complicated... I have people who have decided, have been gone two, three years and after she returned to the violent relationship...."* (Woman social worker, primary care)

Finally, it is important to note that no differences were noted within healthcare level of care, professions, gender, or years of experience regarding opinions of understanding violence against women.

4. Healthcare of Bolivian migrant women

The intersectional approach also highlighted the limits of providers' responses to migration that mainly stress cultural differences between them and migrants or that focus primarily on developing intercultural programs to address cultural barriers.

Among migrants that arrive to health services in Argentina, the Bolivian one appears as "the other" more differentiated, with its own characteristics (language, dress, customs) and phenotypic features, according to providers. Women have a particular weight in the stories of professionals about the Bolivian flow that is largely explained by the type of services analyzed, mainly linked to health. Relationships between migrants and the health system are conflicting as a result of the cultural differences perceived by providers. Cultural differences are mainly related with Bolivian women's traditional figure, associated with submission and docility [37].

> *"In general, the perception of the health team [about Bolivians] is hygiene. It is a main rejection. The other thing is the language. The rhythms are different. They are calmer, more leisurely; they do not ask many questions, or they stay waiting; They do not dare to ask if they need anything. One is very helpless talking but not knowing what happens on the other side."* (Woman gynecologist-obstetrician, third level of care)

> *"The feeling that I have is that they do not have an expression. You do not know if the message was really understood. With an Argentinian woman, it does not happen that much; Argentinian are more questioning, but according to them [Bolivians] everything is always very good."* (Women gynecologist-obstetrician, third level of care)

> *"Those who arrive from there (from Bolivia) have a language that is sometimes difficult to communicate, and they have a deeply rooted culture, the culture they have is very strong. For example, the culture they have is that the husband is the one who transmits everything to his wife."* (Women nurse, third level of care)

> *"The difference (between the Bolivians) with the Argentine ones is the level of education; the Bolivian is submissive, mainly elementary; that is their cultural characteristic; she talks very little and we cannot understand her."* (Women psychologist, third level of care)

Intersectionality analysis contributes to the knowledge offered by existing studies that have sought to understand the relationship of migrant women to health services and have tended to look at the relationship between migrant patients and providers on issues related to communications or cultural interpersonal relations, rather than the simultaneous disadvantages behind the exclusion of certain population groups such as migrant women. In this case, the power of intersectionality approach allows opening the cultural "umbrella" behind opinions and experiences of providers toward Bolivian migrants by enhancing a deeper understanding on how and why this group is looked. It not only shows gender stereotypes (women subject of male domination) but also other social inequalities based on structural roots (such as poverty, xenophobic and discrimination attitudes, ethnic-/race-based discrimination) that shape opinions and experiences of providers toward Bolivian migrants.

Moreover, the lens highlights the importance of taking the migration process as an opportunity to redefine the health-disease-care process in places of migration, placing migrants within the broader contexts where they experience their health. This implies not only focusing on the cultural interpersonal relationships between migrants and providers but recovering the explanations of the multiple causes (cultural, economic, political, social) behind healthcare in migration processes.

5. Conclusions

The findings show the existence of multiple domination systems incorporated in providers' discourses. All of them interact and contribute to gender inequalities in health, specifically on women's access to universal healthcare for violence against women and/or health problems in migrant women increasing their vulnerability. For instance, understanding women as responsible for violence, thinking that violence is a prevalent problem among vulnerable sectors, and conceiving migrants from a solely cultural lens were identified barriers to provide universal healthcare. Working toward universal health coverage is a powerful mechanism for achieving better health and well-being and for promoting human development by ensuring that everyone has access to the health services they need without suffering financial hardship as a result [38].

Intersectionality approach contributed to understand providers' opinions and how in their practices they tended to focus on some factors reproducing inequalities, such as the naturalization of violence against women. In that sense, training and sensitization among providers regarding gender, health, and migration are highly recommended as the first step toward a better healthcare system response and goals defined as improving health and health equity, in ways that are responsive, are financially fair, and make the best, or most efficient, use of available resources [39].

However, it has been pointed that those steps are necessary but not enough to address the multilevel factors shaping healthcare provision [4]. As Thurston and Eisener [40] noted, gender, organizational healthcare culture and structure, and other contextual related variables may play an important role in maintaining barriers and should be studied in depth, avoiding a focus on individual (healthcare provider) level variables.

Therefore, and tacking into account our findings, we propose to question the culture, policies, and practices of the broader structures in which healthcare systems are situated. Opening opportunities to discuss gendered assumptions is essential to promoting gender equity access to health in our context. For instance, this should highlight the importance of taking migrant women's voices to understand how they redefine their understanding of healthcare in their migration process as well as their assets as a way of coping with the multiple obstacles encountered in the health-disease-healthcare at their places of destination. This is why the intersectional approach enhances understanding of inequalities in health and should be strengthened in healthcare policies.

Acknowledgements

The authors are grateful to the participating healthcare professionals and their local health coordinators for their collaboration. Phase two of the project was supported by funds from the Scientific and Technological Research Fund (FONCYT PICT2016-0475). Many thanks to Agostina Ferioli, Fany del Valle Martínez, Elizabeth Viel, Victoria Baudin, Paola Romero, Natalia Funk, Ana Claudia González, and Anahi Rodríguez for their collaboration in phase two of the study. This study was also supported by the Science and Technology Secretary of the National University of Cordoba, Argentina.

Conflict of interest

The authors declared no potential conflicts of interest with respect to the research, authorship, and/or publication of this article.

Author details

Lorena Saletti-Cuesta* and Lila Aizenberg
Culture and Society Research and Study Centre, National Scientific and Technical Research Council, National University of Cordoba (CIECS-CONICET-UNC), Córdoba, Argentina

*Address all correspondence to: lorenasaletti@gmail.com

References

[1] Bowleg L. When black + lesbian + woman ≠ black lesbian woman: The methodological challenges of qualitative and quantitative intersectionality research. Sex Roles. 2008;**59**:312-325. DOI: 10.1007/s11199-008-9400-z

[2] Iyer A, Sen G, Ostlin P. The intersections of gender and class in health status and health care. Global Public Health. 2008;**3**(Suppl 1):13-24. DOI: 10.1080/17441690801892174

[3] Crenshaw K. Demarginalizing the intersection of race and sex: A black feminist critique of antidiscrimination doctrine, feminist theory and antiracist politics. University of Chicago Legal Forum. 1989;**140**:139-167

[4] Kapilashrami A, Hankivsky O. Intersectionality and why it matters to global health. The Lancet. 2018;**391**:2589-2591. DOI: 10.1016/S0140-6736(18)31431-4

[5] Bauer GR. Incorporating intersectionality theory into population health research methodology: Challenges and the potential to advance health equity. Social Science Medicine. 2014;**110**:10-17. DOI: 10.1016/j.socscimed.2014.03.022

[6] Bowleg L. The problem with the phrase "women and minorities": Intersectionality, an important theoretical framework for public health. American Journal of Public Health. 2012;**2**:1267-1273. DOI: 10.2105/AJPH.2012.300750

[7] Shields SA. Gender: An intersectionality perspective. Sex Roles: A Journal of Research. 2008;**59**:301-311. DOI: 10.1007/s11199-008-9501-8

[8] Anderson K. Theorizing gender in intimate partner violence research. Sex Roles. 2005;**52**:853-865. DOI: 10.1007/s11199-005-4204-x

[9] Hunnicutt G. Varieties of patriarchy and violence against women. Resurrecting "patriarchy" as a theoretical tool. Violence Against Women. 2009;**15**:553-573. DOI: 10.1177/1077801208331246

[10] World Health Organization. Prevention of Violence: A Public Health Priority. WHA 49.5. Geneva: World Health Assembly; 1996. pp. 20-25

[11] Kelmendi K. Violence against women: Methodological and ethical issues. Psychology. 2013;**4**:559-565. DOI: 10.4236/psych.2013.47080

[12] García-Moreno C, Hegarty K, Lucas dÓliveira a F, Koziol-McLain J, Colombini M, Feder G. The health-systems response to violence against women. Lancet. 2015;**385**:1567-1579. DOI: 10.1016/S0140-6736(14)61837-7

[13] Montesanti SR, Thurston W. Mapping the role of structural and interpersonal violence in the lives of women: Implications for public health interventions and policy. BMC Women's Health. 2015;**15**:100. DOI: 10.1186/s12905-015-0256-4

[14] García-Moreno C, Jansen H, Ellsberg M, Heise L, Watts C. WHO Multi-Country Study on Women's Health and Domestic Violence Against Women: Initial Results on Prevalence, Health Outcomes and Women's Responses. Geneva: World Health Organization; 2005. p. 206

[15] Plichta SB. Interactions between victims of intimate partner violence against women and the health care system. Trauma, Violence & Abuse. 2007;**8**:226-239. DOI: 10.1177/1524838007301220

[16] Beydoun HA, Beydoun MA, Kaufman JS, Lo B, Zonderman AB. Intimate partner violence against

adult women and its association with major depressive disorder, depressive symptoms and postpartum depression: A systematic review and meta-analysis. Social Science & Medicine. 2012;**75**:959-975

[17] World Health Organization. Strengthening Health Systems to Respond to Women Subjected to Intimate Partner Violence or Sexual Violence: A Manual for Health Managers. Geneva: World Health Organization; 2017. p. 155

[18] Saletti-Cuesta L, Aizenberg L, Ricci-Cabello I. Opinions and experiences of primary healthcare providers regarding violence against women: A systematic review of qualitative studies. Journal of Family Violence. 2018;**33**:405-420. DOI: 10.1007/s10896-018-9971-6

[19] Oso L. La migración Hacia España de Mujeres Jefas de Hogar. Madrid: Instituto de la Mujer; 1998. p. 438

[20] Pessar P, Mahler S. Transnational migration: Bringing gender. International Migration Review. 2003;**37**:812-846

[21] Lugones M. Colonialidad y género. Tabula Rasa. 2008;**9**:73-102

[22] Stolke V. La mujer es puro cuento: La cultura del género. Estudos Feministas. 2004;**12**:77-105. DOI: 10.1590/S0104-026X2004000200005

[23] Donato K, Gabaccia D, Holdaway J, Manalasan M, Pessar P. A glass half full? Gender in migration studies. International Migration Review. 2006;**40**:3-26

[24] Mora L. Las Fronteras de la Vulnerabilidad. Género, Migración y Derechos Sexuales y Reproductivos. Santiago de Chile: UNFPA; 2002

[25] United Nation Fund for Population Activities. Estado de la Población Mundial 2006. Hacia la esperanza, Las Mujeres y la migración Internacional. New York: UNFPA; 2006. p. 116

[26] Martínez-Pizarro J, Reboira-Finardi L. Migración, derechos humanos y salud sexual y reproductiva: Delicada ecuación en las fronteras. Papeles de Población. 2010;**16**:9-29

[27] Cerrutti M. Salud y Migración Internacional: Mujeres Bolivianas en la Argentina. Buenos Aires: PNUD-CENEP/UNFPA; 2011

[28] Aizenberg L, Baeza B. Reproductive health and Bolivian migration in restrictive contexts of access to the health system in Córdoba, Argentina. Health Sociology Review. 2017;**26**:254-265. DOI: 10.1080/14461242.2017.1370971

[29] Braun V, Clarke V. Using thematic analysis in psychology. Qualitative Research Psychology. 2006;**3**:77-101. DOI: 10.1191/1478088706qp063oa

[30] Porto M. Violência contra a mulher e atendimento psicológico: O que pensam os/as gestores/as municipais do SUS. Psicologia: Ciência e Profissão. 2006;**26**:426-439. DOI: 10.1590/S1414-98932006000300007

[31] Heisse L. Violence against women: An integrated, ecological framework. Violence Against Women. 1998;**4**:262-290. DOI: 10.1177/1077801298004003002

[32] Williston CJ, Lafreniere KD. "Holy cow does that ever open up a can of worms": Health care providers 'experiences of inquiring about intimate partner violence. Health Care Women International. 2013;**34**:814-831. DOI: 10.1080/07399332.2013.794460

[33] Thapar-Björkert S, Morgan K. "But sometimes I think . . . They put themselves in the situation": Exploring blame and responsibility

in interpersonal violence. Violence Against Women. 2010;**16**:32-59. DOI: 10.1177/1077801209354374

[34] Sprague S, Madden K, Simunovic N, Godin K, Pham N, Bhandari M, et al. Barriers to screening for intimate partner violence. Women Health. 2012;**52**:587-605. DOI: 10.1080/03630242.2012.690840

[35] Schraiber LB, D'Oliveira AFPL. Romper com a violência contra a mulher: Como lidar desde a perspectiva do campo da saúde. Athenea. 2008;**14**:229-236

[36] Saletti-Cuesta L. Violencia contra las mujeres: Definiciones del personal sanitario en los centros de atención primaria de Córdoba, Argentina [violence against women: Definitions by health professionals at primary care centers in Cordoba, Argentina]. Revista de Salud Pública. 2018;**22**(1):66-76. DOI: 10.31052/1853.1180.v22.n1.17802

[37] Magliano M. Migración, género y desigualdad social. La migración de mujeres bolivianas hacia Argentina. Revista Estudios Feministas. 2009;**17**:349-367. DOI: 10.1590/S0104-026X2009000200004

[38] Dye C, Boerma T, Evans D, Harries A, Lienhardt C, McManus J, et al. Research for Universal Health Coverage. The World Health Report 2013. Geneva: World Health Organization; 2013. p. 168

[39] World Health Organization. Everybody Business: Strengthening Health Systems to Improve Health Outcomes: WHO's Framework for Action. Geneva: World Health Organization; 2007. p. 45

[40] Thurston W, Eisener A. Successful integration and maintenance of screening for domestic violence in the health sector: Moving beyond individual responsibility. Trauma, Violence & Abuse. 2006;**7**:83-92. DOI: 10.1177/1524838005285915

Section 4

Universal Healthcare Cases

Chapter 7

The Brazilian Unified Health System: Thirty Years of Advances and Resistance

Telma Maria Gonçalves Menicucci

Abstract

In 1988, in the context of the re-democratization of Brazil after an authoritarian period, a new Federal Constitution promoted an institutional rupture in the hitherto valid frameworks of health policy, whose origin and expansion until then had been prioritized by the means of insurance restricted to workers inserted in the formal labor market. The constitution has defined principles and guidelines for a reform informed by a publicist perspective and by a conception of health as the right of everyone and the duty of the state, with the corollary of universalization and equality. For this, the unique health system was created. The chapter aims to describe the construction and evolution of the universal health system of Brazil and its results and perspectives. The construction of the universal system from a segmentation legacy, considering the argument that the previous policies defined constraints for the subsequent institutional development, is portrayed. After that, the evolution of the health system and its results and political, financial, and institutional difficulties, also considering the institutional characteristics derived from Brazilian federative institutions, has been discussed. Finally, the country's current political scenario is presented, which points to a new cycle of social policies, including health policy, in the sense of restricting spending and rights.

Keywords: health system, Brazil, universalization, right of the citizen

1. Introduction

After a long period of more than 20 years of authoritarian military governments, in 1988, as a culmination of the country's re-democratization process, a new Federal Constitution was enacted in Brazil. Through this federal constitution, a new political pact was signed not only for the restoration of the rule of law but for a significant expansion of human rights and citizenship, including social rights. Following a trajectory characterized by the structuring and development of a social protection system predominantly corporate-meritocratic, initiated since the 1930s and excluding vast segments of the population, Brazil was in the right step with the pioneer countries that organized welfare systems more robust. And the constitution laid the groundwork for a significant change in both the form of social intervention of the state and the normative and evaluative principles that guide its actions, pointing to a system of universalist protection based on the concept of the right of citizenship.

Among the constitutional changes, it is worth mentioning the introduction of the concept of social security as a more comprehensive form of protection that expresses the idea of the constitution of a network of protection to the social risks inherent to the life cycle, to the labor trajectory, and to the insufficiency of income. In the Brazilian constitutional definition, security comprises an integrated set of actions aimed at ensuring the rights to health, welfare, and social assistance, based on a set of policies with a universal vocation, in addition to expressing an effort to integrate contributory and noncontributory policies based on a broad and diversified funding base.

Particularly in health, the constitutional provisions promoted an institutional rupture in the hitherto valid frameworks of health policy, particularly in relation to health care, whose origin and expansion until then had been prioritized by the means of insurance restricted to workers inserted in the formal labor market. The constitution, which is very detailed in relation to health policy, has defined principles and guidelines for a reform informed by a publicist perspective and by a conception of health as the right of everyone and the duty of the state, with the corollary of universalization and equality. In the 1990s, the process of implementing legal-institutional changes defined in the constitution began, which involved drastic changes in the organization and breadth of the health system. The implementation process was tortuous and conflicting, initially marked by a political, economic, and ideological context, both national and international, not conducive to expansion of spending and state action. However, despite resistance and obstacles, the health policy designed in the constitution was institutionalized, and a universal health system was implemented, with significant results in relation to access, although it is greatly affected by the diverse political and economic conjunctures in which this process has if given, in addition to suffering the feedback effects of previous policies that worked to build a dual system, made up of a public and a private segment.

The recent period, whose results are not yet defined, seems to signal a new cycle of Brazilian social policies in the opposite direction of the Federal Constitution of 1988, in a context of broad political re-articulation and conservative nuance. A broader process of institutional change is under way that signals the reduction of social policies in a context of strong fiscal adjustment and market valuation, in which policies move away from a constitutional normative idea—rights to be guaranteed by the state—and pass to be seen as costs to be reduced due to a supposed exhaustion of funding capacity.

This chapter aims to describe in an analytical way the construction and evolution of the universal health system of Brazil and its results and perspectives. With these objectives, the next section portrays the construction of the system from a segmentation legacy, considering the argument that the previous policies shaped a certain trajectory and defined constraints for the subsequent institutional development, forging, in fact, a dual system, though formally universal. Section 3 discusses the evolution of the health system and its results and political, financial, and institutional difficulties, adding to the analysis the institutional characteristics derived from the format of the Brazilian federative institutions. Finally, Section 4 aligned some conclusions and points out the trends currently that endanger the Brazilian health system.

2. The construction of the universal health system

Assistance to individual health as a public policy was developed in Brazil incorporated into social security benefits and until the Federal Constitution of 1988 was primarily a benefit linked to the formal work contract, not constituting a public benefit to which the entire population is entitled. Another expression of this insurance perspective is the dichotomization that was established in health policy until the end of the 1980s, expressed in a functional and institutional differentiation. The Ministry of Health was responsible for the actions of a collective nature in the form of health campaigns and some basic assistance actions of restricted scope. Social Security, in the various institutional formats that it assumed throughout its trajectory, was the responsibility of individual health care, restricted to the insured and their dependents, which left rural workers and those without a formal employment relationship unprotected. The "regulated citizenship," a conception that expresses the relation between occupation and citizenship, was in force in Brazil, which recognized certain social rights to sectors of urban salaried workers [1]. Among these rights, health care is included, even if secondary to social security benefits.

It was only in the 1960s that there was a substantial expansion of social security health care. This expansion took place largely, particularly in the case of hospital care, through the purchase of services, using the private service network, which developed independently in the public sector [2]. From the 1970s, there was a stagnation in the relative capacity of the public hospital network that remained practically unchanged until the 1990s, which had as counterpart the growth of the importance of the private hospital network[1].

In addition to the purchase of services, another form of articulation between Social Security and the private sector was through the establishment of agreements with companies under which, through a subsidy, the company would assume responsibility for medical care for its employees. In most cases, instead of directly providing the medical services, the company purchased the services of another specialized company, called "group medicine," "medical company," or "medical groups," establishing a triangular agreement between the social security, employer, and medical company. The practice of this covenant favored the expansion of group medicine, restricted to the areas of great concentration of large employer companies, usually located in the more developed regions of the country [4].

Gradually, this form of private health assistance is taking up more space than public assistance in large enterprises on the south/southeast axis—the most developed region of the country—and will be the pillar of the supplementary assistance that will be developed in the following decades.

New forms of inequalities between different strata of workers are introduced in this form of medical care. In general, the agreements were established with large companies, with more specialized labor and higher wages. Medical groups also tend to focus on the more industrialized and urbanized regions. As a consequence, during the 1960s and 1970s, service differentiation would not occur between professional categories but between professional qualifications [5]. Encouraged and legitimized by the public initiative of the agreements, the eminently private forms of health care thereafter developed, which included a great diversity of possibilities of alternative plans and contracts. The different forms of differentiation recreated the particularistic demands of another nature, this time linked to the employment contract and no longer to the professional category.

The counterpart of the option to purchase private health services was the low development of state capacity, mainly for the production of hospital services, which made the public power dependent on the private sector for the expansion of health care. At the same time, the regulatory capacity of the state has not developed, which was strongly captured by private interests. This situation will translate into the prominence of private interests over collective ones, as well as the increase

---

[1] As of the mid-1970s, the number of private hospital beds already corresponded to more than 70% of the country's hospital beds [3].

of the expenses of medical care to levels that would end up compromising the governmental financing capacity of the assistance [4].

A legal instrument, established in the 1980s and in force until today, was the tax waiver that started to function as an indirect state incentive for companies to maintain health plans for their employees. As a result, companies obtained legal permission to pass on their employees' health expenses to product prices, computing health-care expenses as operating costs which is therefore subject to deduction of gross income for the purposes of income tax. Through this indirect incentive, the public decision contributed to the expansion of private health care within companies, already properly structured for this since the 1960s and 1970s, when they had direct incentives.

The same incentive was given to the individual option for private health insurance. The tax policy began to allow deductions of the taxable income of the individuals for the purpose of payment of the income tax and, in this way, contributed to the insertion in the private health insurance or even for the use of the liberal medicine (direct disbursement) of people from the highest income strata. From the point of view of the legitimization of public services, the tax break further weakens the public sector, by favoring the exclusion of its coverage from citizens with greater purchasing power, whose behavior, indirectly, is stimulated by tax policy.

In the 1980s, private assistance ceased to be complementary and became supplementary, becoming autonomous in terms of both funding and how to attract clients. There is a significant expansion of the private forms of health care, both by expanding coverage of business health insurances for service sector workers and of the south/southeast axis and by the autonomous commercialization of health plans due to the migration of clients who paid directly service providers for health insurances as a result of aggressive strategies to expand health insurance markets [6, 7]. By the end of the decade, the private sector was consolidated and quite vigorous.

The worsening of the social security financial crisis in the 1980s marked a moment of inflection, with the emergence of proposals for alternative policies for the health system that emphasized the reversal of the model that privileged private service providers through the channeling of social security resources to the public sector. More or more important than the financial crisis of welfare and the incapacity to sustain this model is the coincidence of the crisis with the process of democratization of the country, which puts on the scene other political actors. In a context of political struggle between alternative health policy projects, it will be possible to change the configuration of the medical assistance model, within the scope, however, of the constraints arising from the institutional configuration of health policy them in force, and whose main features were:

a. The principle of regulated citizenship: health care as a work-related benefit, not as a project of universal and equal inclusion. Parallel to the growth of public health care in a universal sense, the segmentation is recreated through the insertion of some workers in private forms of coverage, favored by public incentives.

b. The option to purchase private services: public assistance is developed through the expansion of the private service network and the atrophy of governmental capacity, both the provider and regulator.

c. The development of a set of private institutions such as group medicine, medical cooperatives, health insurer, and self-management systems (assistance managed by the employer).

d. As one of its consequences, this policy has led to the constitution of a set of institutions and actors and interests. Among the interests constituted, besides the businessmen of the sector, are the beneficiaries of private health insurances, particularly the employees of the companies and public institutions that administer or contract health insurances. By having access to differentiated assistance, they become their supporters, explicitly or implicitly.

In the midst of the country's democratization process, significant changes were enshrined in the new constitution enacted in 1988. The health reform was the result of a broad and victorious political-ideological movement, called the sanitary movement[2], which developed since the mid-1970s, in the context of the authoritarian regime and the struggle for the re-democratization of the country. Opposition to the military regime included the struggle to broaden social policies and redefine them toward universal benefits. The discussion of the "democratization of health" was made more intensely via the "sanitary movement," which achieved a high degree of organicity and great political visibility, and played a relevant role in the reformulation of health policy.

The formation of the health policy reform proposal involved the theoretical construction of a model of understanding the social determinants of health and a set of strategic actions aimed at the dissemination of ideas, the articulation of people and organizations, and the occupation of institutional spaces for experimentation of innovative projects as a mechanism to constitute an alternative to the current policy. Of academic origin, the health reform movement managed to articulate a diverse set of actors, such as the medical category, the "popular health movement," bureaucratic segments, and the municipalist movement, made up of the secretaries and municipal health technicians. One of the political strategies was, on the one hand, to act in the parliament as a place for public debate on health and the organization of the movement and, on the other hand, the involvement with elections of deputies, mayors, and councilors who had health on their electoral platforms and were linked to the more general issue of democratization [8]. In the context of dissatisfaction with the authoritarian regime and in the movement to establish a new pact in the country, it was possible to overcome sectoral or corporate goals and interests in affirming an alternative to the health sector, whose main content was universalization and public responsibility, as opposed to the current segmented and hybrid model.

The new constitutional charter indicated a broad reform in current policy, both in its normative principles and in its organizational format, which significantly altered the previous pattern by breaking with the meritocratic character of health care and incorporating it into the idea of right of citizenship, besides breaking with the previous dichotomization between actions of a collective nature and individual actions. This right to health was defined in the constitution comprehensively as follows:

Article 196. Health is the right of all and the duty of the State, guaranteed by social and economic policies aimed at reducing the risk of disease and other damage and universal and equal access to actions and services for their promotion, protection and recovery.

This definition includes two dimensions. Firstly, the understanding of the social determination of health, indicating that social and economic policies should contribute in reducing the risks of becoming ill, so that the right to health is not limited to access to health services but supposes that all must have the opportunity or appropriate conditions to reach their health potential. Secondly, the definition indicates a public policy guideline for guaranteeing health actions and services,

[2] According to Gerschman, the so-called "sanitary movement" was "a narrow group of intellectuals, physicians and political leaders of the health sector, mostly from the Brazilian Communist Party (PCB), who played a prominent role in opposition to the military regime, as well as a specific political trajectory in the area of health" ([9], p. 41).

guaranteeing universal and equal access to them, expressing a criterion of universal and equal justice in the relationship between the state and citizens.

The focus on the process of implementing the constitutional reform will be equal access to actions and services. In order to give materiality to health policy, the Unified Health System (SUS) was established, defined as the set of public health actions and services provided by federal, state, and municipal public bodies and institutions, since Brazil is a federal state formed by three federative entities with administrative, political, and financial autonomy: the Union, the states (in number of 26), and the municipalities (in number of 5570), besides the federal district constituted by the capital of the country.

The SUS has the following principles: universality of access and gratuity at all levels of health care; equality in care, without any preconceptions or privileges of any kind; the integrality of care, which involves an articulated and continuous set of preventive and curative actions and services, individual and collective; community participation in the process of formulating guidelines and priorities for health policy (by means of health conferences) and in the control and evaluation of actions and services implemented (by means of health councils) at all levels of government; and the political-administrative decentralization, with emphasis on the decentralization of services to the municipalities and the regionalization and hierarchization of the service network.

The SUS funding, defined by the Federal Constitution (FC) of 1988 and amended by the constitutional amendment (CE) in 2000, was defined as the competence of the three federal entities that make up the Brazilian tripartite federation, through resources from its budgets, in addition to including social contributions[3].

As a precursor among developing countries, Brazil was thus establishing, at least from the formal point of view, at the end of the 1990s, a public system of universal coverage defined as an obligation of the Brazilian state. Thus, it preceded what was defined in the WHO Resolution 67/81 on December 12, 2012, which reaffirmed "the right of every human being to the enjoyment of the highest attainable standard of physical and mental health, without distinction as to race, religion, political belief, economic or social condition, and the right of everyone to a standard of living adequate for the health and well-being of oneself and one's family" and recognized "the responsibility of Governments to urgently and significantly scale up efforts to accelerate the transition towards universal access to affordable and quality healthcare services" [10] and to ensure that all people obtain the health services they need without suffering financial hardship when paying for them.

However, the reform of health policy in the late 1980s, which established the universal and public system, failed to incorporate all citizens into free public health care, since some of them were already tied to private forms of assistance. In the constituent process, two opposing visions of health care, defined as "statistic" and "privatizing," were made explicit. If the former represented the innovative perspective of the actors that articulated around the reform, the second represented the interests and conceptions forged in the health policy trajectory as feedback effect of the system in force for more than two decades. Only proponents of the ideas of the health movement had more elaborate proposals, the result of a long process of theoretical development and political articulation. The movement was able to use its knowledge as a power resource in the decision-making process and in the definition of alternatives, making its main proposals reinforced by different categories such as the Central Única dos Trabalhadores (Central Office of Workers), trade

[3] Social contributions in Brazil refer to a specific type of tax destined exclusively for the costing of social security, some of them for social insure costs and others for noncontributory welfare benefits (health and social assistance).

unions of health professionals, and the Council Federal of Medicine, besides part of the members of the constituent assembly. However, the possibility of an abrupt change in the health system based on the universal and public proposal provoked the mobilization and demonstrated the weight and articulation capacity of both representatives of private institutions (group medicine, medical cooperatives, and insurance companies) and private services providers, united in the defense of the pluralism of the forms of health care and of the "freedom of choice." These actors have demonstrated significant veto power, and, although they have not been able to overcome the most significant institutional changes, particularly the creation of a public system of universal access, they have ensured the preservation of previously established arrangements related to private health care [4].

The constitutional text reflected the agreements between these different actors, and its ambiguities reflect the adjustment between innovative alternatives and consolidated standards. The result was the juridical-legal conformation of a hybrid and segmented system that, while, on the one hand, consecrates health as a right, guarantees universality of access to health care, increases state responsibility, and defines the constitution of an inclusive system, on the other hand, preserves market freedom and ensures the continuity of private forms of care, regardless of any governmental intervention.

The change was made possible by an exceptional situation of building a new social pact in the process of democratization and in a situation favorable to institutional imbalances, within the framework of which a new legal framework for health was constituted. Within this framework, it was possible to modify the sectoral political arena with the incorporation of new actors who had alternative proposals, which were confronted with those constituted from previous policies. The public health-care crisis, which translated into widespread dissatisfaction, was another factor that favored institutional change, insofar as the health movement knew how to present an alternative to the crisis, place it on the agenda, and obtain political support for it. In this process, an epistemic community was constituted, whose influence was translated into changes in the political process, because it was able to mediate between the crisis and the choices made and to provide a consistent and widely supported proposal. In the democratic transition, a "political window" was opened, so that the problems of the current policy, associated with the broader political process of democratization, converged in such a way as to allow non-hegemonic political forces to decisively influence the formulation of health policy, giving rise, at a specific moment, to the emergence of a policy informed by a publicist ideology and by a conception of health as a right, having as corollary universalization and equality.

The choices defined in the constitution ensured the continuity of the reform with some degree of continuity, in a process of innovation pressed by interests and objectives that had been constituted as a result of previous policies, which limited the possibility of discontinuous changes but at the same time expressed institutional dynamism when defining a reorganization of the public health system.

3. Implementation and evolution of the health system

In the 1990s, the implementation of health reform began, which included, among other things, the transition from a system that was restricted to salaried workers to a universal system; the decentralization of management to autonomous government units from the political-administrative point of view, replacing a highly centralized model; the unification of previously separated structures and activities (collective actions and individual assistance); the expansion of supply and the reorganization of the health-care model; and the introduction of new management mechanisms that include the participation of society after a long period of restrictions on freedom. This was a major challenge especially for a country with more than 5000 municipalities and deep inequalities between them, both in the capacity to provide services and in socioeconomic conditions and in the health situation and needs [11].

The political conditions for implementing the reform were not very favorable. These include the national and international context marked by the reordering of the role of the state and the state-market relationship in favor of the second and of restriction to universalist policies; the conservative configuration of government coalitions that succeeded the period of democratic transition, in tune with the international environment, which prioritized the processes of adjustment and economic stabilization, accompanied by structural reforms, in the opposite direction to the expansion of government functions and rights enshrined in the constitution; the fragmentation of the health movement and the idealizer of the reform, from the process of democratization, when its heterogeneities and party cleavages were evidenced; the absence of organized support from the main beneficiaries of the SUS, located in the lower social strata; and the fragile and contradictory support of the organized segment of the workers, the majority covered by private health ensures and who did not have immediate interests in a universal system and usually included in their labor agenda the supply of these ensures.

Given the redistributive character of the health reform, broader coalitions would be necessary for its effectiveness, which proved to be very difficult given the political composition of the health arena constituted by different actors and interests configured throughout the health trajectory, as providers of private services, various modalities of health insurance operators, users of private health insurance, etc.

To reach the ultimate goals of the reform, financing was an indispensable resource, involving not only the volume but also the way federal resources were transferred to states and municipalities, since decentralization was made dependent on federal resources. There is a great consensus among analysts and managers in Brazil that financing has been the greatest obstacle to the implementation of the constitutional right to health, but politically the process of its definition has been conflicting, in contexts of restrictive spending policies and lack of definition of sources of financing. After a period of great instability in funding and as a result of pressure from the defense coalition of the SUS, Constitutional Amendment No. 29 was approved in 2000. This amendment defined minimum resources for the financing of public health actions and services in the form of linking budgetary resources of the states and municipalities to health (12 and 15% of their revenues, respectively), and although it established fewer binding rules for the Union, it linked its spending to GDP growth.

Contradictory, in 1998, while discussing the linking of resources to the SUS, the Law 9665 was approved, which regulated private health insurance and plans, and indicated the government's interest in leveraging the growth of the private market. This regulation formalized the duality of the Brazilian health system and politically weakened the proposal of a universal system, although the regulatory process was made independently of national health policy and without even denying or officially redirecting it.

The application of CE 29 has in fact established a sharing between federated entities of health spending and allowed for greater stability in financing, in addition to continuous resource growth, particularly by increasing the expenditures of subnational entities, with a progressive relative decrease in the participation of the Union in the costing of the SUS, although it is still much higher than the expenses of other federated entities (**Table 1**):

	2000	2010	2017
Municipalities	21.7	28.5	31.1
States	18.6	26.4	25.7
Union	59.8	45.1	43.2

Sources: SIOPS/MS [12]; Piola et al., 2018 [13].

Table 1.
Public expenditure on health care by government sphere (%).

However, there is a consensus that resources are insufficient to finance a universal system. In addition to spending relatively little on health (only 6.8% of total public spending and 3.8% of GDP), public health expenditure was US$439.61 in 2014, corresponding to only 46.4% of total spending in health [14]. Pressures for the expansion of resources destined to SUS permeate the history of the sector. A positive response from the National Congress in this regard was the approval of Law 12,858/2013, which included health in the sharing of resources derived from oil royalties, in a context in which the country celebrated the discovery of oil reserves in the pre-salt layer.

Even within a framework of underfunding considering the characteristic of the universality and integrality of the right to health in Brazil, relevant efforts have been made since the 1990s to make these principles a reality. There was, in fact, the implementation of a universal system with a certain standardization of health policy in a country of continental dimensions. This was favored by federal coordination exercised by the federal government, particularly in the form of incentives and regulation of financial transfers, as well as in the form of federative pacts. The SUS is responsible for the vast majority of health services provided in the country and for the total coverage of approximately 75% of the population, since approximately one quarter of it is a beneficiary of private health insurance. In addition, it serves the total population for certain procedures—cases in which the situation of double coverage of citizens with private coverage is characterized since they do not fail to justify universal public service. These procedures include emergency and emergency care, the use of the Mobile Emergency Care Service (SAMU), blood transfusion, transplants, vaccination programs, some high-cost procedures, and, of course, all actions of a collective nature that affect the population as a whole, such as sanitary and epidemiological surveillance. For example, in 2018, the SUS financed more than 11 million hospitalizations and performed more than 3 billion outpatient care [15].

One of the SUS's guidelines is integral care, with priority for preventive activities. Since the 1990s it has been sought to reorganize the care model, seeking to revert the logic of emergency care, generally focused on hospital care, which had characterized health care until then, but with high cost and low effectiveness. To that end, policies and actions were defined, along with financial incentives from the Union to strengthen primary health care more strongly in the 2000s.

SUS is present throughout the Brazilian territory, including isolated indigenous villages and rural settlements, even with regional and local variations due to diverse financial capacity. The distributive and regulatory role of the federal government is fundamental to allow more homogeneity of assistance. The Brazilian public health system is conceived as a federative pact between three government entities and, based on their articulation and cooperation, aims to guarantee the universality and integrality of health care throughout Brazil. Although there is a sharing of functions, the central government concentrates the authority on decision-making process and in the policy regulation, while subnational governments, particularly municipalities, as federated entities with political autonomy, are responsible for

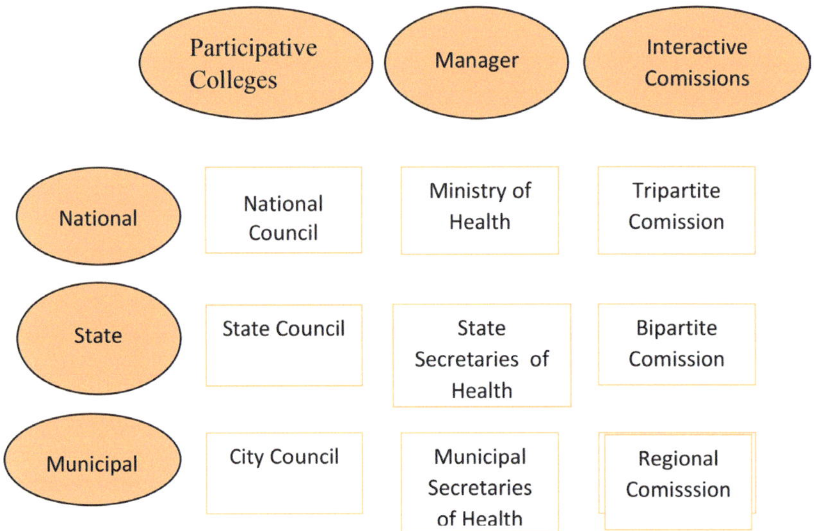

Figure 1.
Institutional and decisional arrangement of SUS. Source: Adapted from Noronha et al., 2008 [16].

policy-making; the states are expected to play the role of coordinating federative pacts between municipalities in their respective jurisdictions and may also be responsible for the provision of more complex services. Institutionalized (tripartite, bipartite regional) committees with normative power aggregate the managers of the different levels of government and are spaces for negotiation and agreement on administrative and financial issues, functioning as federative arenas that articulate the federated entities with shared functions in a national health system organized according to national and binding rules.

It is also worth noting that the participation of society is legally provided by deliberative councils and health conferences, both at the three levels of government. These collegiate instances complete the institutional arrangement of SUS, as illustrated in **Figure 1**.

4. The political turn and the environment of uncertainties: 2015–2019

The materialization of the right to health through the implementation of a universal health system is the result of the post-constitution democratic governments that were challenged to implant SUS, even resistant or facing resistance to the change of status quo. In the 1990s political-institutional advances led toward institutional reorganization, such as the unification of the policy; the construction of the institutional and decision-making framework of the SUS, respecting the federative organization and the social participation guideline; the decentralization and strengthening of municipal health systems; the expansion of actions and services in the national territory; the initial efforts to reorganize the care model with emphasis on primary care; and, at the end of the decade, the definition of new and stable sources of financing. Paradoxically, also at the end of the decade, the regulation of private health plans was formalized, formalizing the dual nature of health care and the cleavage between population covered by private insurance and that covered by the public insurance.

In the twenty-first century, from 2003 to May 2016, Brazil had national governments headed by presidents of the Workers' Party (PT), whose main brand had focused on social policies and the search for reduction of inequalities through development with inclusion. A set of social and economic policies of the period had a potential impact on conditions and health status, acting on the first dimension of the right to health defined in FC 1988. The fight against hunger and misery deserved special attention, including income transfer programs and agrarian development policy, besides fight against racism and racial inequalities, constitution of social assistance policy, growth of the social security coverage rate through measures aimed at reducing informal work, implementation of an urban development policy, and recovery of minimum wage values.

However, starting in 2015, one of the country's biggest political and institutional crises begins, with strong repercussions on the future of Brazilian social policies, including health policy. President Dilma Rousseff from the start of her second term in 2015 had the subject of a strong campaign for her removal and the target of an oppositional attack that manifested by the total boycott of her government and the government's capacity. Started by the party that lost the elections (PSDB), the impeachment movement of the newly elected president gained supporters among sectors and more conservative parties, business sectors, and part of the middle class. The signs of an economic crisis and the unraveling of investigations into corruption in the state-owned Petrobras company that reached the political support base of the government provided ammunition for the opposition, strongly supported by the mainstream media, that managed to mobilize significant sectors of the population from the motto of the fight against corruption, leading to the gradual loss of government support and popularity. In the midst of this movement, and articulated to it, the public sphere began to express conservative Government Proposals and restrictions on state action, in clear opposition to the policies developed in the last two decades in the country.

The outcome of this process was the removal of the president, provisionally in May and definitely on August 31, 2016, after a process that observed the constitution in rites and procedures but was quite debatable in its substance to not be able to unambiguously characterize a crime of responsibility of the president, which would provide the constitutional justification for its deposition. Vice-president Michel Temer assumes the government—active articulator of the process of impeachment—with a large majority in the congress and with proposals for deep and structural reforms, both in the economic area and in social and labor policies and in the field of foreign policy. An accelerated process of constitutional change and the deconstruction of the status quo begin under the cloak of severe fiscal adjustment and "modernization," with a cut in public expenditures, privatizations, and threats to social policies capable of rendering ineffective rights enshrined in the constitution.

Regarding health policy, specifically with regard to its financing, some decisions, on the one hand, indicate restrictions on the financing of the SUS and, on the other hand, signify changes in the principles on which the health system is based. These include:

a. Establishment of the *new fiscal regime*, which aims to establish, for 20 years, ceilings for primary expenses (excluding interest payments) within the Union, which are limited to the variation of the inflation index as measured by the Extended National Consumer Price Index (IPCA) and based on 2016 expenses; this ceiling mitigates the binding nature of constitutionally defined health expenditures and affects all social policies.

b. Government Proposals to strengthen and expand private health insurance, justified by the need to "rethink" constitutional rights such as universal access to health, on the grounds that the country is supposed to be unable to support them anymore. These proposals were translated into the creation of an "affordable health insurance" with a lower cost and a list of services lower than the mandatory minimum established by the National Agency of Supplementary Health (ANS), as well as proposals for changes in the regulation of the supplementary health sector, very favorable to the operators, to the detriment of the users.

c. Changes in the format of intergovernmental relations, with a reduction in the role of federal coordination by the federal government.

The recent agenda thus points to the underfunding of the SUS, deregulation of the system with reduction of federal coordination, and expansion of the private sector with less regulation. It foresees a new health reform "inside" and without fanfare, which without denying the SUS will make it systemic if it is implemented [17].

It is beyond the scope of this article to analyze the political-institutional crisis in Brazil that began in 2015, but I would like to emphasize here one of its effects which was the intensification of political cleavages, which had many consequences, particularly in the electoral process. Firstly, it prevented the country's main popular leader from running for the 2018 presidential elections, arrested on charges of corruption that were not proven materially and from a highly questionable legal process both nationally and internationally. Secondly, the crisis allowed the victory of an extreme right-wing politician who proclaimed in discourse the deconstruction for the construction of a new country and that has as economic minister a radical liberal, supported by business sectors that give support to the new government.

The current period may represent the beginning of a new cycle whose contours are delineated, but whose results are still unpredictable. Democracy also seems threatened in one of its foundations which is a guarantee of social rights which has the utopia of greater substantive equality, beyond legal-formal equality, as one of its foundations. It is worth remembering that the concept of social policy has become inseparable from the notion of citizenship, which implies the establishment of a set of rights and duties between the citizen and the state and, fundamentally, the recognition of equality among citizens. It is, therefore, an egalitarian notion that relates to the construction of democracy—a political system based on the assumption of a basic equality among citizens. But even in democratic contexts, social policies tend to be subject to normative controversies involving conceptions of the role of the state and of justice. In the last decades, a great debate about these rights has been experienced in a context of persistent and widespread economic crisis. On one side, there are some interpretations, which emphasize the cost of social policies and consider the maintenance of these rights unsustainable, on the other hand, in different visions, social policies are seen as investment and producers of a more just and sustainable development, especially in countries which have not yet reached adequate levels of development.

In Brazil today, the first vision prevails in the government sphere and the attack against social policies, and the rights they represent are not an isolated event, but are linked to a set of governmental decisions and actions that form a coherent and articulated whole that points to changes in the way the Brazilian state operates, which directly affects social policies. Instead of isolated actions, we have actions that are concatenated with a view to redirect the interventionist or more proactive state standard (both with measures aimed at the development of the economy and at mitigating the perverse effects of the market economy) toward a market society with few state moorings. This would translate not only into more visible processes such as privatizations, sale of public assets, outsourcing, and incentives to market development in areas traditionally attributed to the state, such as health, but in deregulation processes (in various fields). Among these, the reform of labor legislation that has already been implemented is a great example of considerably reducing state regulation of the relationship between the employer and employee in a situation of great disparity in bargaining power due to high unemployment rates, which in practice allows and accentuates the suspension of guarantees established in previous legislation. This reform tends to increase worker informality and instability, and this outcome, in turn, should have an impact on the very sustainability of social security (which is also the subject of a reform proposal), as more precarious employment ties will have negative effects on the collection of social and pension contributions by workers and companies and, therefore, in the financing part of the social policies in force.

The commemoration of the 30 years of the Brazilian constitution, dubbed as "citizen constitution" for the rights it enshrines, among them the right to health, coexists with an ongoing process of deconstruction or of a larger institutional change in which the association between economic and social development, which was the hallmark of previous governments, loses strength in the current political conjuncture, as well as the proactive role of the state in this regard. Although the developments in this process are not given yet, the current period signals a new cycle of social policies in the opposite direction of the Federal Constitution of 1988.

If the right to health implies a state guarantee of the adoption of public policies that avoid the risk of harm to health, considering all the health determinants, such as healthy environment, income, work, sanitation, food, and education, as well as the guarantee of health services that promote, protect, and recover individual and collective health, the Brazilian future does not seem promising. In all of these areas, there is an institutional deconstruction in Brazil, which includes cutting resources and changing legislation in the sense of social deprotection and market favoring in the context of an exacerbated and authoritarian liberalism. In the case of health, after three decades of building a universal and integral system, it is predicted that the system will be exhausted, even if it is not programmatically denied; it can suffer from a systemic unfeasibility that could lead to its degradation.

Author details

Telma Maria Gonçalves Menicucci
Federal University of Minas Gerais, Belo Horizonte, Brazil

*Address all correspondence to: tgmenicucci@gmail.com

References

[1] dos Santos WG. Cidadania e Justiça (Citizenship and Justice). Rio de Janeiro: Campos; 1979

[2] Braga JC, Paula SG. Saúde e Previdência: Estudos de Política Social (Health and Welfare: Social Policy studiEs). São Paulo: Cebes Hucitec; 1981

[3] Brazilian Institute of Geography and Statistics (IBGE). Health Statistics—Pesquisa de Assistência Médica-Sanitária (Survey of Medical-Health Care); 1999

[4] Menicucci Telma MG. Público e Privado na Política de Assistência à Saúde no Brasil: Atores, Processos e Trajetória (Public and Private Health Care Policy in Brazil: Actors, Processes and Trajectory). Rio de Janeiro: Fiocruz; 2007

[5] Giffoni RM. Público e Privado na Política de Assistência à Saúde no Brasil: Atores, Processos e Trajetória (Medical Assistance and Work Relationships in the Company: The Model of Agreement with Social Security) [Master's dissertation]. São Paulo: University of São Paulo; 1991

[6] Faveret PF, Oliveira PJ. A universalização excludente: Reflexões sobre as tendências do Sistema de Saúde (the exclusionary universalization: Reflections on the trends of the health system). DADOS-Revista de Ciências Sociais. 1990;**33**(2):257-283

[7] Bahia L. Planos e Seguros Saúde: Padrões e Mudanças das Relações Entre o Público e o Privado no Brasil (Plans and Health Insurance: Patterns and Changes in Public-Private Relations in Brazil) [Doctoral thesis]. Rio de Janeiro: National School of Public Health, Oswaldo Cruz Foundation; 1999

[8] Rodrigues Neto EE. A via do parlamento (The way of the parliament). In: Fleury S, editor. Saúde e Democracia: A Luta Do CEBES (Health and Democracy: The Struggle of CEBES). São Paulo: Lemos Editorial; 1997

[9] Gerschman S. A Democracia Inconclusa: Um Estudo da Reforma Sanitária Brasileira (The Unfinished Democracy: A Study of Brazilian Sanitary Reform). Rio de Janeiro: Fiocruz Publishing House; 1995

[10] World Health Organization. Resolution Adopted by the General Assembly. 2012. Available from: https://www.un.org/en/ga/search/view_doc.asp?symbol=A/RES/67/81

[11] Menicucci T. A Relação Entre o Público-Privado e o Contexto Federativo Do SUS: Uma análise Institucional (The Relation Between The Public-Private and The Federative Context of SUS: An Institutional Analysis). Series Social Policies. Vol. 196. Santiago: CEPAL; 2014

[12] SIOPS/MS. Health Information System/Ministry of Health

[13] Piola SF, Benevidesm RPS, Vieira FS. Consolidação Do Gasto Com Ações e Serviços Públicos de Saúde: Trajetória e Percalços no Período de 2003 a 2017 (Consolidation of Spending on Public Health Actions and Services: Trajectory and Mishaps in the Period from 2003 to 2017). Text for Discussion 2439. Rio de Janeiro: IPEA; 2018

[14] Figueiredo JO, Prado NMBL, Medina MG, Paim JS. Gastos Público e Privado Com Saúde no Brasil e Países Selecionados (Public and Private Health Expenditures in Brazil and Selected Countries). Health Debate; Rio de Janeiro. Vol. 42, Special Issue 22018. pp. 37-47

[15] DATASUS. SUS Department of Informatics. Ministry of Health

[16] Noronha JC, Lima LD, Machado CV. O sistema único de saúde—SUS (The unified health system—SUS). In:

Giovanella L, Escorel S, Lobato LVC, Noronha JC, Carvalho AI, editors. Políticas e Sistema de Saúde no Brasil. (Policies and Health System in Brazil). Rio de Janeiro: Fiocruz Publishing House; 2008

[17] Telma M. Política de saúde do Brasil: Continuidades e inovações (Health policy in Brazil: Continuities and innovations). In: Arretche M, Marques E, Faria CA, editors. As Políticas Da Política: Desigualdades e Inclusão Nos Governos Do PSDB e Do PT (Policy' Politics: Inequalities and Inclusion in the Governments of the PSDB and PT). No press; 2019

Chapter 8

Economic Crisis, Decentralisation and Health Inequalities: The Case of Italy

Stefano Neri

Abstract

The chapter describes the recent evolution of the Italian National Health Service (NHS), highlighting the potential and effective consequences of the economic and financial crisis on social and territorial inequalities, especially in terms of service access and quality. First, it analyses the cost-containment and austerity policies in the NHS, which brought to a relevant underfunding of the public healthcare system, comparing public expenditure trends in Italy with those of other Western European countries. Then, it stresses the increasing role played by private expenditure, emphasizing the risks in terms of health inequalities connected to the high level of out-of-pocket payments and to the spread of the occupational funds. Finally, a reconstruction and analysis of the current changes in the NHS governance is carried out, explaining in details how the reassertion of the role of the Central State in health policy entails different consequences for different areas of Italy, widening the territorial inequalities and increasing the North-South divide. So far, these changes have taken place without any structural reform, in an imperceptible but progressive way, which does not help to develop an appropriate and necessary debate on the future of the healthcare system.

Keywords: healthcare, decentralisation, national health service, health inequalities, economic crisis

1. Introduction

Since the Italian unification (1861), the Italian healthcare system has fully changed its institutional model at least three times. From being substantially 'residual' during the liberal era (1861–1921) and also the fascist decades (1922–1943), with a gradual spread of corporate health funds and some compulsory insurance schemes targeted on specific illnesses [1], it shifted to a social health insurance system at the end of the fascism, which was developed after the end of the Second World War, during the first 30 years of the Republic (1945–1977); finally, an universalist National Health Service (NHS) was instituted in 1978 (Law no. 833). Structural changes were then adopted in 1992–1993 (Legislative Decrees no. 502/1992 and no. 517/1993), introducing managerialisation and managed competition, which was softened in 1999 (Legislative Decree no. 229/1999), while Constitutional Law no. 3/2001 recognised, at constitutional level, and strengthened the regionalisation of the healthcare system carried out during the 1990s [2].

IntechOpen

As a result, the NHS is structured on three levels: a national level, constituted mainly by the Ministry of Health; an intermediate level represented by the Regions and their Regional Ministers and health departments and a local operational level, directly accountable to the Regional one, made up of about 70–75 *Aziende sanitarie ospedaliere* (hospital trusts, henceforth HTs) and about 135–140 *Aziende sanitarie locali* (local health authorities, henceforth LHAs).

Since 2001, no major reforms have been introduced into the NHS. However, important changes have almost imperceptibly taken place, connected the economic and financial crisis, which are weakening the universalist nature of the NHS.

This chapter will analyse the evolution of the NHS in Italy during the last decade, hence in the years of the crisis, focusing on some trajectories of change underway, mainly in the health expenditure and in the NHS institutional framework governance. These trends might have important consequences in terms of service access and quality, increasing the traditional social and territorial inequalities and hence weakening the universalistic nature of the NHS.

2. What universalism? NHS performance between North and South

According to international and national literature, the Italian NHS system performs relatively well in comparative terms, among both European and OECD countries, although it is questionable whether and to what extent some of the results reported in the adopted indicators are attributable to the healthcare system in itself. The OECD report *Health at a Glance* [3], which represents a systematic evaluation of the healthcare systems in 35 OECD countries, based on 76 indicators gathered in 9 categories or areas (health status, risk factors, access to care, quality of care and health outcomes, health expenditure, staff, care provision, pharmaceuticals, ageing and long-term care), the OECD *Health profile* on Italy [4] and the OECD/EU report *Health at a Glance: Europe 2018* all agree attributing, by and large, good results in terms of prevention, access and quality of care, mortality and survival rates as well as in terms of health expenditure and efficiency, with improvements in many areas compared with the beginning of the 2000s. However, as emerged not only by OECD reports but also by other literature, social inequalities are significant in many indicators related to dimensions such as health status, risk factors, access and quality of care [3–9].

In particular:

- From 2000 to 2015, life expectancy at birth has increased from 79.9 to 82.7 years (the second best figure in the EU after Spain), thanks mostly to the decrease of the mortality for cardiovascular diseases. However, there are relevant gender and social inequalities.

- As far as risk factors are concerned, from 2000 to 2014, the rate of smokers has decreased from 25 to 20% slightly below the EU average. Also obesity rates decreased, but they remain considerably high, especially among children, with 18% of children aged 7–8 years in condition of obesity in 2017 (the second highest level in Europe, 6 points over the EU average).

- Coverage rates for several types of immunisation are at the level of the comparable European countries, although they have slightly decreased after 2012–2013 (but it is expected to have increased again in most recent years in the case of children vaccinations). Conversely, rates of cancer screening have increased [6].

- Avoidable mortality (preventable and amenable) is one of the lowest in Europe, and also survival rates for different types of cancer and major cardio-circulatory illnesses are within the average or among the best found among Western European comparable countries.

- In terms of access, the Italian NHS provides coverage to all citizens and foreign residents with a comprehensive care based on health needs, but social and territorial inequalities are relevant.

- In 2017, health expenditure was below the EU average, both in terms of per capita expenditure (2,551 Euro, −8.1% compared with the average EU level) and of share of the GDP (8.9, −0.6% compared with EU average). Although the NHS ensures a wide package of free services, out-of-pocket expenditure (23% of total health expenditure in 2015) is much higher than the EU average (15% in 2015).

- Long-term care is still lacking, with several indicators below the level of Western European comparable countries, although there are signs of improvements in the last years.

However, as it is well known by NHS scholars, national figures reported in international statistics and comparisons hide the very relevant differences existing among different areas of countries, traditionally summarised in the North-South divide. In this respect, 1992–1993 reforms had introduced the 'Livelli Essenziali di Assistenza' (essential levels of healthcare), or LEAs, which include all the kinds of healthcare services to be provided by all the regions throughout the country. Every year Central State attributes to regions the amount of funds needed to the provision of this very wide service package, after a State-Regions negotiation based on an allocation defined according to per capita criteria, adjusted for the distribution of the population by age and epidemiological factors.

The LEAs, which were first released in 2001, are matched with a monitoring and control system based on a set of indicators which allow checking whether and to what extent regions are respecting and ensuring the LEAs in the healthcare service provision to their resident population. The indicators are grouped in three areas of healthcare (prevention; outpatient, community and home care; hospital care). For each area, a synthetic index is obtained from the relevant indicators, with scores which may vary between 0.00 and 100.0 points. The monitoring system is associated to incentives and sanctions in terms of attributed funds.

Last assessment carried out by the Ministry of Health in 2017 [10] showed the persistence of very relevant disparities among Regions, with Northern Regions nearly always having the best scores in most of the indicators of the three areas of healthcare. Moreover, differences in the scores are striking, going, in prevention, from 80.92/100.00 points by Lombardy to 48.48 by Sicily; in outpatient care, from 86.39/100.00 by Liguria to 29.05 by Campania and in hospital care, from 89.13/100.00 points by Tuscany to 25.41/100.00 points obtained by Campania. Although many indicators are focused on expenditure efficiency, they highlight also the very important territorial differences existing in terms of service access and quality, in favour of Northern and Centre-Northern Regions.

These differences are historically rooted. However, despite significant efforts especially addressed to reduce territorial differences in expenditure for health services [11], these were not translated into a correspondent reduction of the differences existing in terms of service quality and efficiency between different areas of the country. Quite the opposite, according to some studies, the North-South gap has been widened since the 1990s, that is, in the years of NHS regionalisation, instead of being reduced [12–14].

In this context, the economic crisis started in 2008–2009 triggered a set of policies which, on the one hand, risk to deepen the existing social inequalities in terms of service access; on the other hand, they caused a substantial change in the NHS governance which could seriously increase the territorial differences.

3. The economic crisis and austerity policies in the NHS

In Italy, the economic crisis started in 2008 was prolonged, with a fluctuating trend, characterised by two peaks (**Table 1**): the first was in 2008 and especially in 2009, when the Italian GDP declined by 1.1 and 5.5%, respectively, from the previous year. After an overall weak recovery in the following 2 years, in 2012, the crisis heightened and the GDP dropped by 2.8%, followed by a further decline of 1.7% in 2013. In 2014–2015, the GDP growth trend was very slack and became a little more sustained in 2016–2017 (respectively, 1.1 and 1.6%), but in 2018, it dropped down again below 1%, and also provisional data for 2019 indicate a further weakening of the economic recovery (Eurostat database). In all these years, the GDP growth rates were considerably lower than those of the 28 EU countries (**Table 1**). Similar differences emerge also considering only the countries within the Euro area.

The recession had a very strong impact on the relationship between the GDP and public debt. Since 1991–1992, this ratio had always been at more than 100%, one of the highest in Europe, except for 2007 (99.8%). However, since the start of the economic crisis, it has progressively increased surpassing the 130% of the GDP in 2014, with a tendency to level off over this level (**Table 2**).

Beyond the data, the crisis became particularly serious in 2011–2012, when the widespread perception, by the international markets and European institutions, that the Italian government was no longer able to bring the debt under control resulted in a sovereign debt crisis. This brought to the fall of the Berlusconi government, at the end of 2011, replaced by a 'technical' executive, headed by the economist Mario Monti. In the context of a protracted financial crisis and lack of confidence of the international environment, strict austerity measures were taken to control the budget deficit, reduce public sector expenses and increase public revenues [15]. While in policy areas such as pensions, these measures were accompanied by structural reforms; this was not the case in healthcare which was, however, object of severe cost-containment and retrenchment measures.

In the Italian highly regionalised NHS, control of health expenditure by the central government was pursued primarily through extremely limited increases, and, in some cases, reductions in the level of funding are attributed by the central government to the regions to finance the LEAs. The level of annual funding of LEAs is calculated in the budget laws, called 'stability laws', and it is negotiated between the State and the Regions within the State-Region Conference (see below) and

	2007	2008	2009	2010	2011	2012	2013	2014	2015	2016	2017	2018
Italy	1.5	−1.1	−5.5	1.7	0.6	−2.8	−1.7	0.1	0.9	1.1	1.6	0.9
Eu 28	3.1	0.5	-4.3	2.1	1.8	−0.4	0.3	1.8	2.3	2	2.4	2.0

Source: Eurostat: National accounts and GDP online database.

Table 1.
GDP rates: percentage change on previous year.

ratified in official acts and documents such as the 'State-Region Agreements' or the 'Pacts for Health'. However, the Parliament and the central government can modify the concerted funding levels, as has always occurred in fact, after the beginning of the crisis with reductions in the originally agreed funds.

Absolute values and percentages of annual funding increases confirmed a stagnation in the central government financing from 2010 onwards, with very reduced surges but also drops compared with the previous years, in 2013 and in 2015 (**Table 3**). From 2010 to 2019, central funding increased by about 8,800,000,000 Euro, with a yearly average of about 0.9%, less than the average yearly inflation rate (about 1.1%; see [16, 17]).

Besides the containment of general central funding, austerity policies addressed the control of specific sources of expenditure arising from the acquisition of production inputs. The main cost-containment programmes started in 2009 (Law Decree No. 39/2009) and 2010 (Law Decree No. 78/2010) and intensified in the following years, culminating in the so-called spending review on public administration, promoted by the Monti government in 2012 (Law Decree No. 95/2012, converted into Law No. 131/2012). The austerity measures then continued roughly until at least 2016, albeit with less intensity, and the cost-containment in healthcare remains one of the central government priorities.

Main policies included spending caps and reduction in the pharmaceutical expenditure; decrease in hospitalisation rates and in the number of hospital beds per

2007	2008	2009	2010	2011	2012	2013	2014	2015	2016	2017	2018
99.8	102.4	112.5	115.4	116.5	123.4	129	131.8	131.6	131.4	131.2	131.4

Source: Eurostat: General government gross debt online database.

Table 2.
General government gross debt in Italy: percentage of GDP.

	Financing (in Euro)*	Change compared with previous year (in Euro)*	Change compared with previous year (%)
2007	97,600,000,000	(4,400,000,000)	(4.7)
2008	101,600,000,000	4,000,000,000	4.1
2009	104,200,000,000	2,600,000,000	2.6
2010	105,600,000,000	1,400,000,000	1.3
2011	106,900,000,000	1,300,000,000	1.2
2012	108,000,000,000	1,100,000,000	1.0
2013	107,000,000,000	−1,000,000,000	0.9
2014	109,900,000,000	2,700,000,000	2.7
2015	109,700,000,000	−200,000,000	−0.2
2016	111,000,000,000	1,300,000,000	1.2
2017	112,600,000,000	1,600,000,000	1.4
2018	113,400,000,000	800,000,000	0.7
2019	114,400,000,000	1,000,000,000	0.9

**Approximate.*
Source: Ministero della Salute [16].

Table 3.
Financing of the central funding for LEAs.

1000 inhabitants; a redefinition, in a generally restrictive sense, of the criteria used to set the regional tariffs (linked to DRG-like systems), for inpatient and outpatient services provided to the NHS; general restrictions of the expenditure on purchases of goods and services; increasing revenues, mainly by increasing the copayments for citizens, although Regions have the possibility to make partially different choices.

These measures were added to those aimed at controlling staff expenditure in all public services [15], which are of particular significance due to the importance of human resources in the health sector. In the NHS there were main two types of measures addressed to public providers: measures aimed at gradually reducing the number of employees and others at containing wage and salaries.

In the first case, at the end of 2006, and thus before the start of the crisis, a cap for personnel expenditure in the NHS, which had to be equal to the 'corresponding amount of the year 2004 reduced by 1.4%', including costs for temporary employees and autonomous workers. This measure has been substantially confirmed, with some minor changes, until May 2019, when it was replaced by less restrictive constraints.

A predictable result of the cap and other similar measures was a slowdown and substantial stop in the staff hiring and turnover within the NHS healthcare organisations. Between 2008 and 2017, the staff of the NHS passed from 689,873 to 647,048 total employees, a drop of 42,825 employees (−6.2%; data taken from the Ministry of Economy and Finance online database). The decrease was highly significant, considering that the Italian healthcare service is understaffed compared with many European countries [1].

Staff hiring was reopened in 2017–2018; especially after that the new national NHS collective agreement signed in 2018 opened the possibility to hold extraordinary public competitions for the new recruitment of doctors, nurses and technical health personnel. These measures were confirmed by the stability law for 2019. However, the pace of recruitment seems inadequate to face the lack of healthcare staff within the NHS, which will become more serious in the next years considering the predictable wave of retirements connected to an ageing labour force, especially among doctors [18].

Furthermore, a second type of measures concerned the containment of wages for employees in the NHS, as well as independent professionals working for the NHS, starting from the general practitioners and paediatricians. After moderate wage increases in 2008–2009, national-level collective bargaining was suspended for 2 years, in 2010, for all 2,800,000 contractualised public employees, including NHS staff. The suspension was then extended until 2015, when a sentence of the Constitutional Court forced the government to restart the collective bargaining process in the public sector. A new national NHS collective agreement for the period of 2016–2018 was signed in May 2018, with modest pay increases. Collective negotiations at decentralised level was not frozen but was put under strict financial constraints, with the prohibition to exceed the amount of resources used in 2010. The overall effect of these provisions was to freeze the salaries of NHS employees for 8 years, substantially to the levels of 2010.

In addition to these measures, there were also specific measures addressing the Regions in conditions of high deficit in the health sector and therefore subjected to a recovery plan, which will be dealt in the second part of the article.

4. Dynamics of public and private expenditure: out-of-pocket payments and occupational funds

The overall effect of the austerity policies and public underfinancing policies has been a recalibration in the health expenditure levels, which were already lower than the average values recorded in comparable continental and Northern European countries, and in line with the other countries of Southern Europe (in particular Spain and Portugal). In Italy, in 2015–2016, the total health expenditure in fact amounted to 8.9–9% of the GDP (+0.7–0.8% compared with 2007), two points (or more) below than in France, Germany and Sweden, which traditionally have expenditures higher than Italy, and also nearly a point less than in the UK, which has always been a very parsimonious country. In 2017–2018, the total health expenditure amounted to 8.8% of the GDP (OECD database).

Also public (or government) health expenditure is lower than in the main continental and Northern European countries, in terms of both the share of the GDP and per capita expenditure (**Table 3**). Starting from a precrisis value of 6.3% (2007), the Italian government expenditure, GDP ratio did not grow even by half a percent in the following decade (6.6% in 2017 and 6.5% in 2018 estimation), despite the inevitable increase in demand for services with a steadily ageing population, which has the highest share of the over 60 age bracket in Europe (22.3% in 2017) and the highest median age in Europe along with Germany (45.9 in 2017, Eurostat database). Similarly, public expenditure per capita on health services increased by 18% from 2007 to 2018, a share much lower than in the main continental and Northern Europe countries reported in **Table 4**.

Italian trends in public expenditure on health are more similar to those of other Mediterranean European countries such as Portugal and Spain, although, from 2007 to 2016, the growth of expenditure per capita in Spain was certainly higher (23.3%).

At the same time, the share of private health expenditure over the total expenditure on health, while diminishing in France, Germany and Sweden, increased in the UK, Italy and other Southern European countries (**Table 5**). In Italy, from 2007 to 2018, it shifted from 22.5 to 25.8% of the total health expenditure, therefore coming to represent more than a quarter of total health expenditure. This brought the level of private health expenditure closer to that of Spain. Highest ratios of private health expenditures, which should not be typical of NHS systems, are shared by other Mediterranean countries such as Portugal and Spain (and, of course, Greece where private health expenditures represent nearly 40% of total health expenditure).

The increase in private health expenditure, traditionally high, entails serious risks of worsening in social inequalities, in an era of economic crisis, especially because in Italy it is mainly constituted by out-of-pocket payments which, as it is well-known, emphasise the role of socioeconomic inequalities in service access. Between 2007

	Share of GDP (%)			Per capita (US$PPP)			Growth of expenditure per capita (%)
	2000	2007	2018p	2000	2007	2018p	2007-2018p
France	7.6	8.0	9.3	2119	2770	4141	33.1
Germany	7.7	7.5	9.5	2260	2809	5056	44.4
Sweden	6.3	6.6	9.3	1878	2647	4570	42.1
UK	4.7	6.1	7.5	1238	2111	3139	32.7
Italy	5.5	6.3	6.5	1474	2088	2545	18.0
Portugal	5.9	6.2	6.0	1127	1548	1902	18.6
Spain	4.9	5.7	6.2	1087	1795	2341	23.3

p = provisional value. Source: OECD Health Care online database.

Table 4.
Levels of current public expenditure on healthcare.

and 2014, the share of individuals reported unmet needs for medical examinations (because they were too expensive, because care facilities were too far away or because of waiting lists) for medical examinations shifted from 4.1 to 7.0%, highly concentrated in the share of population with the lowest income (elaborations by E. Pavolini on OECD health care online database). It is quite likely that the combination between cost-containment and retrenchment policies in the public sector and the increase in the role of private expenditure played an important role in determining this result.

However, an important part of the growth of private health expenditure in Italy during the crisis was due to the insurance component. In this regard, one of the most recent transformations that has taken place in Italy in relation to private health expenditure is the spread of occupational health funds for workers and their families, introduced or reintroduced from national collective bargaining or unilateral initiatives by employers (**Table 6**).

Although the occupational funds were almost non-existent in the 1990s, they have increased dramatically in the past decade, especially since the mid-2000s, reaching more than 10,000,000 people, around 33–35% of the total employees, in 2017. Most of the workers registered to an occupational scheme are employees (63% of total registered people), which mostly belong to the private sector, given that occupational schemes in healthcare are still nearly absent in the public sector.

The increased role of occupational healthcare funds represents a major challenge to the universalistic nature of the Italian NHS for three main reasons [19]: (a) they are increasingly financing core healthcare provision (especially diagnostics

	2007	2018p	Diff 2018p-2007
France	22.9 (9.5)	16.6 (9.4pp)	−6.3 (−0.1pp)
Germany	24.9 (14.3)	15.5 (12.3)	−9.4 (−2.0)
Sweden	18.1 (16.9)	16.1 (14.8)	−2.0 (-2.1)
UK	18.3 (10.4)	20.5 (16.0pp)	2.2 (5.6pp)
Italy	22.5 (21.5)	25.8 (23.1)	3.3 (1.8)
Portugal	31.3 (25.7)	33.5 (27.4pp)	2.2 (1.9pp)
Spain	27.3 (21.0)	29.5 (23.6pp)	2.2 (2.6pp)

p = provisional value; pp = data referred to 2017. Source: OECD Health Care online database.

Table 5.
Private and out-of-pocket health expenditure in share of total health expenditure (%) (in brackets: out-of-pocket health expenditure as % of total health expenditure).

Categories	No. of registered people to occupational schemes	%
Employees	6,692,000	63.0
Independent workers	1,062,239	10.0
Employee relatives	1,944,634	18.3
Independent workers relatives	216,070	2.0
Pensioners and relatives	500,966	4.7
Pensioner relatives	200,386	1.9
Total	10,616,847	100.0

Source: GIMBE [17], elaborated from data by the Ministry of Health.

Table 6.
Registered people to occupational schemes: 2017.

and ambulatory care), which should be offered by the NHS, acting as a substitute for NHS services rather than completing or supplementing them; (b) access to occupational healthcare funds is profoundly affected by the employees' occupation and their position in the labour market (fixed-term vs. open-ended contracts, manual occupations vs. nonmanual occupations, unskilled occupations vs. skilled professions, etc.), and coverage is therefore rather unevenly distributed among workers and also in relation to the sector of employment; and (c) occupational schemes are concentrated among workers employed in big and medium-sized firms; this entails the creation of inequalities among those employed in firms of different sizes. Moreover, as medium and big firms are mainly located in the North of Italy, the spread of occupational funds brings serious risk to deepen the traditional differences existing in service access and quality between the North and the South of the country.

5. The evolution of the governance of the NHS between the reassertion of the role of the State and the development of a differentiated regionalism

Unlike the oldest national health services, such as those of England or Sweden, the Italian NHS has always had a decentralised structure, in line with the Italian Constitution. In a first phase (1978–1992), the powers and responsibilities were divided among the State, Regions and local government. With the reforms of 1992–1993 (Legislative Decrees No. 502/1992 and No. 517/1993), instead, the regionalisation of the NHS was introduced, together with its managerialisation [5, 20]. Regionalisation was then strengthened by the Constitutional reform introduced in 2001 and confirmed by the failures of subsequent attempts of Constitutional reforms in 2006 and 2016.

According to current regulation, legislative powers are shared between Central State and Regions. As already mentioned, the State is in charge of defining the 'essential levels of healthcare', or LEAs, and has to guarantee regions the financial resources necessary for LEA provision. Regions and the two Autonomous Provinces of Trento and Bolzano have great freedom in organisation and management of their Regional Health Services. Starting from the second half of the 1990s, different 'regional healthcare models' emerged, characterised by regulatory structures marked by hierarchical integration, cooperation or competition between purchasers and service providers [2]. NHS regionalisation includes also a certain degree of fiscal autonomy, even if very restricted (see [21]), as well as the possibility of introducing copayments for drugs and outpatient services at regional level.

The balance of powers between state and regions that emerged from the regionalisation introduced during the 1990s and in 2001 required a permanent mechanism of negotiation and, possibly, cooperation between the State and the Regions to define national health policy.

On the one hand, since 2001 the central government has been *de facto* unable to implement institutional and organisational reforms without the consent and the involvement of regions. On the other hand, regions must respect a national regulative framework which imposes significant constraints on their possibility to introduce institutional changes within the regional healthcare systems. Therefore, concerted policy-making has been developing since 2000–2001. It has given rise to a series of 'agreements', 'pacts' or 'ententes' signed in the 'State, Regions and Local Governments Conference' (simply called State-Regions Conference) and then converted into legislation by the Parliament.

The State-Regions Conference includes the Prime Minister as President of the Conference, the Presidents (or Governors) of the Regions or other Ministers whenever matters related to areas of their competence are discussed. Instituted in 1988 and strengthened in 1997, in the first part of the 2000s, the Conference came to play a major role in national healthcare policy-making, representing the main institutional mechanism able to ensure close cooperation among Regions and permanent negotiation between those and the central government (see [22] for more details).

Although none of the regulatory changes had modified the above-described division of powers, the economic and financial crisis as well as political responses to the crisis weakened the role of the regions in national policy-making, in favour of greater importance of the role played by the central government, the Ministry of Economy and Finance (MEF) and, indirectly, by the European institutions. State-Region Conference has partially lost its centrality in policy-making, given that concerted policy-making has been increasingly substituted by unilateral decision-making by central government and supra-national institutions.

This shift became particularly evident after the explosion of the sovereign debt crisis of 2011–2012. The need to take urgent measures able to signal to international markets and the EU the willingness and ability of the national Government to bring the public debt under control have prompted approval of measures, contained in the laws of stability and austerity packages adopted by the Central Government, which in great part had not been agreed upon and basically not even discussed with the regions, Parliament and organised interests. The minimisation of room for discussion and negotiation was motivated by the lack of time and alternatives in the face of the commitments made with the EU and the need to reassure the markets. These dynamics did not occur only in Italy but were common to all the European countries most affected by the financial crisis and sovereign debt, namely, those of Southern Europe and, in a partially different form, Ireland [23–26].

The reassertion of the role of the State was enhanced by the economic crisis, but it had already started before 2007–2008. In the mid-2000s, many Regions showed to be unable to control health expenditure growth and contain regional deficits. In order to ensure compliance with the European Stability and Growth Pact, in 2005, the central government and Regions agreed on a multistep mechanism of regional expenditure monitoring and recovery plans in the case of excessive deficits. If a Region accumulates serious deficits and misses spending targets, the agreement provides for the activation of automatic mechanisms (like an increase in regional taxes) and the close supervision of regional expenditure policies by the MEF. Central government may appoint a commissioner in charge of NHS administration in that Region and impose specific measures to reduce deficits, thereby introducing severe limitations on regional autonomy.

To date, the recovery plan mechanism has been activated in 10 (out of 20) regions, and 5 of them have been subjected to administration by a commissioner. In 2019, seven regions are subject to a recovery plan; most of them entered the mechanism between 2007 and 2010. These regions include all Southern and Southern-Central Regions except the small Basilicata, while only two Northern Regions were forced to approve a recovery plan and were never commissioned.

Despite differences between individual cases, the recovery plan mechanism was largely effective in securing a debt reduction of the regions. The success was such as to cause the Government to introduce a control mechanism of deficits of individual NHS providers, bound to the presentation of plans, in 2015.

However, experience has shown that, once the plan procedures began, it was extremely difficult to abandon them. This was due not only to the presence of particularly demanding financial targets in years of economic crisis but also to the existence of objectives beyond purely economic aspects that impacted on quality and access to services. In many cases these objectives were not easy to meet, considering that recovery plans inevitably required retrenchment policies which entailed severe cuts and other kind of restrictions in service provision. On this respect, this monitoring mechanism might have determined a worsening in some dimensions linked to access and service quality, widening the gap between Southern Regions which entered into the recovery plans and Northern Regions free from the plans and their constraints.

From the point of view of the intergovernmental relations, the recovery plan mechanism severely restricted the autonomy of regional governments in the development of health policies. Central government and, in particular, the MEF not only exerted a penetrating supervision and monitoring of the plan implementations in the regions concerned but also, often, gained the right to exert a sort of veto, in the face of regional policies that involve increased expenditure. Although the formal division of powers between the levels of government has not changed over the past decade, regional decentralisation proved in fact to be much weakened in favour of an increase of the Central State's regulatory role, embodied by MEF rather than by the Ministry of Health [27, 28].

If Central and Southern-Central healthcare have been subjected to these strict forms of control during the years of crisis and until now, this has not been the case of the Northern and Central-Northern regions, except for two cases (Piedmont and Liguria). In most of these regions, the ability to maintain fiscal equilibrium or limited deficit has allowed them to consolidate the autonomy of regional health policies, even in the presence of nationally determined austerity policies.

Moreover, some of these regions (Emilia-Romagna, Lombardy and Veneto) have formally demanded 'further forms and conditions of autonomy' (Article 116, cl. 3, Italian Constitution), both in the health sector and in other policy sectors, which would make them more similar to the five Italian regions provided, from the 1950s, with a special autonomy for historical or ethnical reasons.

After the successful consultative referendum held in Lombardy and Veneto on 22–23 October 2017, and the formal request of the Emilia-Romagna government between August and October 2017, a negotiating table was opened with the central government, according to the procedure laid down in Art. 116 of the Constitution. Although negotiations are still underway, with serious conflicts emerged between the two parties of the current coalition government, it is quite clear that the request of more autonomy should concern not only the management of resources but also regional tax capacity, so as to take a significant step towards a more complete accountability of the regions. One of the most delicate issue concerns the possibility to retain most of fiscal revenues collected within any single region, limiting the process of central redistribution. Given the very relevant differences in fiscal capacity between the North and the South of Italy, the potential effects of this change could be highly detrimental for Southern Regions.

6. Conclusions

Economic and financial crises which severely hit Italy did not result into structural and fundamental changes in the NHS. However, it prompted or accelerated some processes which seriously risk to gradually change a universalist healthcare system into a more hybrid one. Retrenchment and austerity policies in the public, underfinanced NHS find some sort of compensation in the high level of private out-of-pocket expenditure and in the spread of occupational funds. As a consequence, traditional inequalities in access to healthcare services are deepening and seem bound to increase, exacerbating differences among socioeconomic and occupational groups.

Moreover, the trend to informal but substantial re-centralisation in national policy-making, with the reassertion of the role of the state in charge of playing the role of 'financial watchdog' of regional governments, is having different consequences for Northern and Southern Regions. The former was able to retain their autonomy, so that to develop health policies targeted to the needs of their citizens, while the ladder entered into a monitoring mechanism of their expenditure, which is giving significant results in financial terms but risk to worsen service access and quality.

So far, healthcare system 'hybridisation' [29] and the trend to 'differentiated federalism' [28] or 'differentiated autonomy' have occurred without any structural reforms, by means of imperceptible but progressive changes which, in terms of institutional change, may be qualified in terms of 'gradual transformation' [30, 31]. However, the formal request for constitutional change by three regions and related, current political conflicts, as well as the increasing complaints and also protests by doctors and healthcare experts on NHS underfinancing, emphasised by the media, might help promote an open debate on the future of the Italian NHS and health policy, which has been completely lacking so far.

Author details

Stefano Neri
Department of Social and Political Sciences, University of Milan, Italy

*Address all correspondence to: stefano.neri@unimi.it

References

[1] Vicarelli G. Healthcare: Difficult paths of reform. In: Ascoli U, Pavolini E, editors. The Italian Welfare State in a European Perspective. Bristol: Policy Press; 2015. pp. 157-178

[2] Neri S. The evolution of regional health services and the new governance of the NHS in Italy. In: Douglas A, Zoe B, editors. Health Studies: Economic, Management and Policy. Athens: Atiner; 2011. pp. 269-282

[3] OECD. Health at a Glance—OECD Indicators. Paris: OECD Publishing; 2017. Available from: http://www.oecd.org/health/health-systems/health-at-a-glance-19991312.htm

[4] OECD. Italy: Country Health Profile 2017. Paris: OECD Publishing; 2017. Available from: http://www.oecd.org/fr/italie/italy-country-health-profile-2017-9789264283428-en.htm

[5] Giarelli G. 1978-2918: quarant'anni dopo. Il Ssn tra definanziamento, aziendalizzazione e regionalizzazione. Autonomie Locali e Servizi Sociali. 2017;**3**:455-482

[6] GIMBE. Il Servizio Sanitario Nazionale nelle classifiche internazionali. In: Report Osservatorio GIMBE 4/2018. Fondazione GIMBE; 2018. Available from: https://www.gimbe.org/pagine/1207/it/report-42018-il-ssn-nelle-classifiche-internazionali

[7] OECD/EU. Health at a Glance: Europe 2018: State of Health in the EU Cycle. Paris: OECD Publishing; 2018. DOI: 10.1787/health_glance_eur-2018-en

[8] Sarti S, Terraneo M, Tognetti Bordogna M. Poverty and private health expenditures in Italian households during the recent crisis. Health Policy. 2017;**121**(3):307-314

[9] Terraneo M. La salute negata. Le sfide dell'equità in prospettiva sociologica. Milano: Franco Angeli; 2018

[10] Ministero della Salute. Monitoraggio dei LEA attraverso la cd. Griglia LEA. Metodologia e risultati dell'anno 2017. Roma. 2018

[11] Mapelli V. Il sistema sanitario italiano. Bologna: Il Mulino; 2012 (new edition)

[12] Pavolini E, Vicarelli G. Is decentralization good for your health? Transformations in the Italian NHS. Current Sociology. 2012;**60**(4):472-488

[13] Toth F. How health care regionalisation in Italy is widening the North-South gap. Health Economics, Policy and Law. 2014;**9**(3):231-249

[14] Toth F. The Italian NHS, the public/private sector mix and the disparities in access to healthcare. Global Social Welfare. 2016;**3**:171-178

[15] Bordogna L, Neri S. Austerity policies, social dialogue and public services, in Italian local government. Transfer: European Review of Labour and Research. 2014;**20**(3):357-371

[16] Ministero della Salute. Il finanziamento del Servizio Sanitario Nazionale. 2019. Available from: http://www.salute.gov.it/portale/temi/p2_6.jsp?id=4752&area=programmazioneSanitariaLea&menu=dati

[17] GIMBE. 4° Rapporto sulla sostenibilità del Servizio Sanitario Nazionale. Fondazione GIMBE; 2019. Available from: http://www.rapportogimbe.it/

[18] Vicarelli G, Pavolini E. Health workforce governance in Italy. Health Policy. 2015;**119**(12):1606-1612

[19] Arlotti M, Ascoli U, Pavolini E. Une transformation structurelle en cours dans le système de santè italien: les fonds de santé. In: Ferréol G, editor. Systèmes de santé et politique de soins: vers de nouveaux défis? Louvain-la-Neuve: EME; 2018. pp. 193-208

[20] France G, Taroni F. The evolution of health-policy making in Italy. Journal of Health Politics, Policy and Law. 2005;**30**(1-2):69-188

[21] Bordignon M, Mapelli V, Turati G. Can we fit a square object in a round hole? Fiscal federalism and national health service in the Italian system of governments. In: ISAE, Annual Report on Monitoring Italy, Rome. 2002. pp. 37-125

[22] Maino F, Neri S. Explaining welfare reforms in Italy between economy and politics: External constraints and endogenous dynamics. Social Policy & Administration. 2011;**45**(4):445-464

[23] Asensio M, Popic T. Portuguese healthcare reforms in the context of crisis: External pressure or domestic choice? Social Policy & Administration. 2019;**1**:1-15. Available from: https://onlinelibrary.wiley.com/doi/epdf/10.1111/spol.12480

[24] Pavolini E, Guillén AM, editors. Health Care Systems in Europe Under Austerity: Institutional Reforms and Performance. Basingstoke: Palgrave; 2013

[25] Pavolini E, Lèon M, Guillén AM, Ranci C. From austerity to permanent strain? Comparative European Politics. 2015;**13**(1):56-76

[26] Sotiropoulos DA. Southern European governments and public bureaucracies in the context of economic crisis. European Journal of Social Security. 2015;(2):226-245

[27] Frisina-Doëtter L, Neri S. Redéfinir le rôle de l'État dans le soins de santé: une analyse comparative de l'Italie et des États-Unis. In: Ferréol G, editor. Systèmes de santé et politiques de soins: vers de noveaux défis? Louvain-la Neuve: EME Éditions; 2018. pp. 175-191

[28] Frisina-Doëtter L, Neri S. Redefining the state in health care policy in Italy and the United States. European Policy Analysis. 2018;**4**:234-254

[29] Rothgang H, Cacace M, Frisina L, Grimmeisen S, Schmid A, Wendt C. The State and Healthcare: Comparing OECD Countries. Houndmills: Palgrave Macmillan; 2010

[30] Streeck W, Thelen K, editors. Beyond Continuity. Institutional Change in Advanced Political Economies. Oxford: Oxford University Press; 2005

[31] Neri S. The Italian NHS after the economic crisis: From decentralization to differentiated federalism. e-cadernos CES. forthcoming